Alzheimer's Disease

Alzheimer's Disease

PREVENTION, INTERVENTION, AND TREATMENT

Elwood Cohen, M.D.

KEATS PUBLISHING

LOS ANGELES

NTC/Contemporary Publishing Group

Library of Congress Cataloging-in-Publication Data
Cohen, Elwood.
    Alzheimer's disease : prevention, intervention and treatment / by
Elwood Cohen.
        p.   cm.
    Includes bibliographical references and index.
    ISBN 0-87983-964-3 (pbk.)
    1. Alzheimer's disease Popular works.   I. Title.
RC523.2.C64   99-10314
616.8'31—dc21   CIP

Published by Keats, a division of NTC/Contemporary
Publishing Group, Inc.
4255 West Touhy Avenue
Lincolnwood, Illinois 60646-1975 U.S.A.

Design by Robert S. Tinnon

Printed and bound in the United States of America
International Standard Book Number: 0-87983-964-3
10 9 8 7 6 5 4 3 2 1

Contents

This book is dedicated to Hazel Wooten,

a regal soul whose journey might have been eased

had today's advances been known in the early years.

Acknowledgments

I would like to acknowledge my wife and children for their encouragement, which helped bring this book to fruition. Particular thanks go to our son Craig, whose exemplary computer literacy and patience saved me from years of frustration on a computer full of glitches and unending crashes, and from a keyboard that seemed forever bereft of letters. Special thanks go to our daughter Brandi for her computer skills and readiness to come to my rescue on so many occasions.

I would like to acknowledge my mother for her encouragement over the past years and to congratulate her for ninety years of a productive and continued fruitful life.

I would like to thank Mr. Merwin Snyder for contributing his invaluable suggestions, assistance, and encouragement leading to publication of this book.

I would like to thank Professor Tom Hersh at Orange Coast College for leading me out of the depths of computer illiteracy, for his invaluable training in teaching me to utilize the Internet for research, and for his immeasurable assistance.

I would like to thank Dr. David Kaufman for his exemplary research assistance.

I would like to thank Ms. Jeanette Mahoney for her great assistance and kindness in extending her skills to make this book a success.

I would like to thank Dr. Shirley Gaffey for her invaluable literary advice and assistance, and her encouragement in getting this book in the hands of our distinguished publisher.

I would like to thank Dr. Roberta Gladstone for her clinical excellence, sincerity, and empathy with patients, for her review of the manuscript, and for her encouragement and gracious collaboration in the psychiatric aspects of Alzheimer's disease.

I would like to thank Dr. Jack Florin, whose admirable prowess in neurology and profound dedication to medicine command the exceptional respect he receives from his colleagues, for his superb critique of the manuscript, and for his assistance in getting this book to press.

I would like to thank Dr. Marvin Gladstone, who possesses an extraordinary command of family practice medicine and a profound lifetime devotion to his patients, for his masterly critique of the manuscript and most valuable suggestions.

I would like to thank Dr. John Kirby, whose expertise and advice in radiology, magnetic resonance imaging, and advanced scanning procedures translate masterfully to the diagnosis of Alzheimer's disease. His conscientious review of the manuscript and assistance with this book have proven invaluable.

I would like to thank Dr. Rod St. Clair for his exceptional prowess in internal medicine and acute understanding of Alzheimer's disease and related dementias. His conscientious, in-depth review of the manuscript and superb advice in all aspects has greatly helped to make this book a success.

I would like to thank Dr. Jane Xenos for her timely assistance, for the enlightenment into her field of expertise, for her pioneering efforts in the emerging field of craniosacral therapy, and for her wisdom that physical medicine is an integral and indispensable part of general medicine.

I would like to thank all of the medical specialists for their professional prowess, sincerity, uncompromising efforts, and exemplary care they have provided to so many of my lovely patients over the past several years. No one can tally the lost hours of their lives sacrificed to weekend and middle-of-the-night pilgrimages to our area emergency rooms. They and their colleagues are a dying breed; I shall remain forever indebted to them. It has truly been said of acute-care providers that their wives are widows and their children are orphans.

I would like to thank Dr. Hazem Chehabi for his invaluable expertise and assistance with PET scans and his acute vision of their future role in the diagnosis of Alzheimer's disease.

I would like to thank Ms. Nancy Kolodny, editor at Keats Publishing, for her superb literary talent, kindness, expediency, and knowledge.

I would like to thank Mr. Tom Hirsch, editor at Keats Publishing, for his initial evaluation of this book, his astute recognition of its merits, and his exceptional help and advice.

I would like to laud in particular those innumerable, beautiful Alzheimer families everywhere for their undying efforts, unselfish patience, and the years of their lives freely given to provide exemplary care to their loved ones. Their paths have not been easy. Their personal sacrifices are resolute. They deserve far greater recognition than I am humbly able to provide.

I would like to thank Richard Gallen, whose wisdom and foresight were responsible for launching this book.

Foreword

The term "Alzheimer's disease" carries with it the connotation of fear and death. Those who have closely encountered it recognize that the dementia ushers in a slow downward spiral from the loss of memory, to detrimental personality changes, and finally to the progressive depletion of motor controls and body functions. Those family members who become the caregivers can expect to pay an exacting toll in the demands upon physical strength and in the hours of sleep deprivation. They experience a myriad of emotional traumas that are often more painful than those suffered by the patient.

The disease process follows a progressive downhill course. The patient regresses as family members helplessly observe one year after another disappear from their loved one's memory as the patient's mind meanders backward through childhood. Consternation envelops family members as they become increasingly concerned with their own risk of inheriting the same dementia. Their distress is understandable.

Until recently, the disease was one about which very little was known and for which there was little to offer therapeutically, save exemplary caregiving. But a metamorphosis in our knowledge has occurred within the last five years. To better understand this disease, recognize its symptoms, and seek proper help, we need only to look in medical textbooks, contact Alzheimer's assistance organizations, and become involved with Alzheimer's discussion groups. For those of us familiar with computers, there is an abundance of help accessible from both the World Wide Web and Internet. Any physician can provide you with in-depth descriptions. The Alzheimer's Association has a wealth of information available as do local libraries. There are over 500 books in print with titles relating to Alzheimer's disease.

The emotional shock of observing the disease as it engulfs a loved one is a normal reaction. It is a bitter pill for anyone to swallow, no matter how well prepared physically and emotionally we think we are . Families and friends experience the kind of trauma that a diagnosis of an incurable cancer with prolonged duration would trigger. It has been difficult to advise that there is no cure, that there is little help, that the disease is a progressive death sentence.

In order to arrest any disease, four elements of a quadrangle must be recognized: symptoms, causes, diagnosis, and treatment.

As far as Alzheimer's is concerned, only symptoms have been recognized, and even then they have been initially overlooked. All four legs of the quadrangle will be needed for truly effective prevention and this has not yet fully transpired. However, the requirements are rapidly being met. Dramatic advances in diagnostic modalities, laboratory tests, and cognitive testing allow doctors to detect the disease much earlier than was possible years ago, and this means we can now take steps to intervene clinically, long before marked and irreversible brain damage takes place.

There are also little-known but excellent markers for the disease. One example is that fingerprint patterns are significantly predictive of Alzheimer's disease years before its onset, just like a fold in an earlobe denotes an early predictive feature for heart attacks. Other early markers involve such areas as decreased sensorial levels and pre-dementia depression. These changes show up years before perceptual symptoms of Alzheimer's surface and give us focal points to begin strategies.

Much the same as with any disease, a diagnosis is required so that appropriate treatment can be administered. Alzheimer's can exist in a pure state by itself or in combination with other dementias that can mimic it. It has been difficult to differentiate Alzheimer's from other related dementias, and at times, nearly impossible to separate it from mixed types of dementia. Alzheimer's has been referred to as a "diagnosis of exclusion." Historically, the only definitive diagnosis has been by autopsy. Newer diagnostic tests are in developmental stages that will have an accuracy approaching that of autopsy. Moreover, these procedures herald a much earlier diagnosis. Before prevention can be effected, however, the other two legs of the quadrangle are still required: causes and treatment.

Our emerging knowledge about Alzheimer's causes provides us with greater understanding about the pathogenesis of the disease. We are now aware of several causes that are totally avoidable, such as head trauma, thiamine deficiency, estrogen deficiency, and certain medications. Many causes can be blocked by preventing the progression of their deleterious effects in the brain.

Approximately 20 percent of Alzheimer's cases are genetically oriented. Several genes have been identified as mutants. The age of onset of symptoms is usually sixty-five and older, and these are recognized as including both familial and sporadic varieties. The younger the onset of symptoms occurs, the greater the likelihood of genetic mutation. There is also a maternal link to an increased incidence of Alzheimer's. The other 80 percent of cases are due to a variety of causes; some are known, such as low blood sugar, trauma, and nutritional deficiencies, but most still remain unknown.

Happily we have made quantum leaps forward with earlier

identification of symptoms, greater recognition of causes and their pathological brain changes, and much earlier diagnoses. This enables us to embark on the fourth leg of the quadrangle: treatment and prevention. Near-miraculous strides in treatment enable doctors to retard the progression of Alzheimer's, slowing even advanced cases. Early intervention is the essential key to preventing the disease process.

For example, there are a number of agents capable of retarding progression of the inflammatory and abnormal metabolic changes that take place in the brain. We must rely upon more than one agent to achieve measurable protection against progressive brain damage, inevitable dementia, and death. Although mild megadosing of medicines in the face of multiple causes of the disease is presently required, there are negligible side effects.

There are, at present, several classes of medications in the research stage, designed so that they provide a range of patient responses, from symptomatic relief to total arrest of the disease process. Eventually, one or two medicines may emerge to control the disease and prevent the ravages of Alzheimer's. However, we would be terribly remiss to overlook the treatments presently available in favor of awaiting the eventual arrival of a monotherapy (single medication). The prudent course is to utilize the proven agents at hand. To that end, a protocol of treatment is presented here to prevent Alzheimer's, and it has been pared down to the most crucial ingredients. Although the number of medicinal agents recommended is the minimum required in the treatment plan, others are carefully explained and can be incorporated into the protocol to stimulate even greater response.

This book offers a treatment plan gleaned from the latest research and clinical experience for achieving dramatic results in the fight against Alzheimer's disease. Many of the causes will come as a surprise. Other cornerstones of ancillary treatment such as caregiving, avoidance, and diet and nutrition are included along with medicinal protocols.

Finally, this book attempts to present Alzheimer's as it really is! It bares the symptoms from subtle to severe, upgrades our ability to diagnose the disease long before symptoms become obvious, and offers strategies by which physician and family, working together, can better treat and eventually prevent the disease.

CHAPTER 1

Preview: Fifty Revealing Facts About Alzheimer's

As a quick, educational primer, here is a valuable list of fifty pertinent facts about Alzheimer's.

Fact #1. There are over 4 million Americans suffering with Alzheimer's. The number will increase to 14 million people in the next generation or two. There are 20 million Americans directly affected by it, and this will progress to 70 million.

Fact #2. The combined expenses to treat Alzheimer's in the United States exceed $100 billion annually.

Fact #3. Approximately 50 percent of the population will develop Alzheimer's if they survive past the age of eighty-five.

Fact #4. Twenty percent of all Alzheimer's cases are related to genetic inheritance.

Fact #5. Alzheimer's can be prevented. Even moderately advanced stages can be delayed. Early recognition is the key to treatment and prevention.

Fact #6. The larger the brain, the greater the reserve that remains throughout the course of this developing dementia. Larger brains show better performance during the downhill spiral of Alzheimer's.

Fact #7. It is now generally accepted that the course of Alzheimer's disease might start as early as the fetal stage and will intermittently traverse several decades. It can have slow and sporadic periods of development, as well as acute phases, depending upon the underlying causes, the individual's physiologic status, and genetic mutations.

Fact #8. Short-term memory loss is the most prominent early symptom of Alzheimer's. It can be very subtle in onset, and initially it is cleverly hidden by the patient.

Fact #9. Little-known fingerprint patterns can predict the development of Alzheimer's years before its clinical onset, and with such accuracy that they have been proven an excellent marker. A simple home test will reveal it.

Fact #10. The sense of smell is lost approximately two years prior to other symptoms. It is an early marker for disease. Its onset is so gradual over such a prolonged period of time that the patient is often totally unaware. Simple home testing can expose it.

Fact #11. Hearing loss is extraordinarily high in Alzheimer's and occurs earlier than other symptoms. It is an early marker for identifying disease and easy to detect.

Fact #12. Depression is a very early marker. It is encountered in 50 percent of all patients suffering with dementias. In Alzheimer's, its onset is seen earlier than other dementias, setting it apart from them. It can present itself more than two years before the disease is recognized.

Fact #13. Survival is generally six to eight years after diagnosis. However, death can occur as soon as two years after the diagnosis has been established.

Fact #14. Seventy percent of all deaths due to dementias are of the Alzheimer's type. There are many other dementias that mimic Alzheimer's, of which vascular dementia is the most frequently encountered.

Fact #15. Individuals with low blood sugar (hypoglycemia) have nearly twice the chance of developing Alzheimer's dementia because their brain cells are deprived of the sugar required for energy and survival.

Fact #16. Diabetics have only one-half the risk of developing Alzheimer's disease.

Fact #17. Prolonged psychological stress can induce Alzheimer's.

Fact #18. Prolonged use of the antihistamine type of nerve medicine, chlorpromazine (Thorazine), can contribute to Alzheimer's disease.

Fact #19. Prolonged use of stomach medicines such as Donnatal and Bentyl might play a significant role in causing, or at least aggravating, Alzheimer's.

Fact #20. Electromagnetic fields are now implicated as a cause of Alzheimer's.

Fact #21. Exposure to several groups of organic solvents such as toluene is implicated as a possible cause of Alzheimer's.

Fact #22. Several anti-inflammatory agents such as ibuprofen are able to reduce the risk of developing Alzheimer's as much as 55 to 60 percent by their ability to counteract the inflammatory processes in the brain that are responsible for the death of brain cells that cause Alzheimer's.

Fact #23. Shingles, a very painful skin rash caused by a virus, can produce a dementia identical to Alzheimer's.

Fact #24. Autopsy reveals that Alzheimer's patients are deficient in thiamine (vitamin B_1). Correcting this deficiency with vitamin supplements has been shown to improve cognition.

Fact #25. Estrogen replacement therapy provides a 55 percent reduction in the risk of developing Alzheimer's disease.

Fact #26. Aluminum has been alleged to be a major cause of Alzheimer's disease.

Fact #27. Zinc is now a primary suspect among the heavy metals suspected as a potential cause of Alzheimer's.

Fact #28. Iron deposits in the brain are prominent in Alzheimer's and may possibly evolve as a cause of dementia.

Fact #29. The lack of circulation with a corresponding loss of oxygen and glucose (sugar) to the brain is highly suspected to be a contributing cause of Alzheimer's disease, even as early as the fetal stage.

Fact #30. Children of affected mothers have a significantly higher rate of Alzheimer's (9:1) compared to children of affected fathers.

Fact #31. Several genes have been identified that cause Alzheimer's, and the earlier its onset the more likely the cause is genetic.

Fact #32. Apolipoprotein E 4 (APOE 4) is a harmful inherited gene, carried by 30 percent of the population, but fortunately only 10 percent of those who carry it will ever develop Alzheimer's.

Fact #33. Head trauma, particularly accompanied by loss of consciousness, doubles the risk of Alzheimer's. Head trauma with possession of the abnormal hereditary gene APOE 4 increases the risk of Alzheimer's tenfold.

Fact #34. Alzheimer's dementia has been documented in individuals as young as age twenty-nine, representing an inherited genetic subset of the disease.

Fact #35. The Cherokee Nation of Native Americans exhibits a natural immunity to Alzheimer's.

Fact #36. African-Americans and Hispanics are both at higher risk than whites for developing Alzheimer's.

Fact #37. AD 7 C has to date proven to be a most significant test and it closely matches autopsy findings for diagnostic accuracy.

Fact #38. The PET scan is unique for measuring blood flow and metabolism in the brain. It is reported to have the potential to predict Alzheimer's as many as twenty years before clinical symptoms evolve.

Fact #39. Nicotine improves learning and slows the progression of Alzheimer's, although this is not an excuse for smoking.

Fact #40. Vitamin E is 55 percent effective against Alzheimer's. It can help to prevent the disease if started early in the course of treatment.

Fact #41. Haldol, a nerve medicine initially marketed for the treatment of schizophrenia and other psychoses and now used for other nervous disorders, can significantly retard the progression of Alzheimer's.

Fact #42. Certain ulcer medications such as Tagamet provide significant delay in both onset and progression of Alzheimer's.

Fact #43. Fish oils (omega-3) are protective against Alzheimer's and help prevent depression.

Fact #44. Levels of vitamin B_{12} normally decrease with aging, but Alzheimer's patients have lower levels of vitamin B_{12} than their normal counterparts and this deficiency requires replacement.

Fact #45. Ginkgo biloba is an herb with many beneficial properties and it can delay the progression of Alzheimer's. It is a mainstay of treatment worldwide.

Fact #46. Sundowner's syndrome refers to wandering and roaming when the sun goes down. Melatonin may help to alleviate sundowner's syndrome and help regulate and normalize sleep patterns.

Fact #47. Gotu kola, an herbal medicine known as a longevity drug in China, increases mental acuity, improves circulation, and helps alleviate sundowner's syndrome.

Fact #48. Epileptic-type seizures can be a very early marker of a rare genetic subset of Alzheimer's and can occur even before the early onset of disease at ages as early as twenty-nine.

Fact #49. St. John's wort is an herbal medicine used very successfully over many centuries for the treatment of depression. It is reputed to be as effective as Prozac, without side effects, available without prescription, and much less expensive.

Fact #50. Transplanting cells from the testicle of one species into the brain of another species is a current research project designed to improve cognition in Alzheimer's patients.

These fifty facts represent only a small part of the current knowledge about Alzheimer's disease and are elaborated throughout the following chapters. They are presented here in chapter one to familiarize you with the many important new discoveries relating to this elusive disease. The purpose is to introduce a medical background to enable the reader to gain insight into the complexity of Alzheimer's. We are about to embark on a continuum of exciting advances that will catapult this once-hopeless disease into a realm of newly evolving treatments. Step by step, we will travel through the course of this disease onto a stratum of protection and prevention. There is so very much that can be done at present, and the future is bright with promise of additional success.

CHAPTER 2

Overview

Alzheimer's disease has been referred to as both the plague of the ages and the plague of the aged. This disease was so poorly understood that people who suffered this dementia were labeled as tormented, affected, pixilated, weird, afflicted, senile, mad, crazy, and spellbound. They were feared, avoided, ignored, and ridiculed. Over the centuries they suffered terrible and inhuman treatment when their families hid them away from public view, restrained them at home, incarcerated them in locked rooms, and committed them to insane asylums. Some were believed possessed by demons, others were accused of witchcraft, and as recently as two centuries ago were even burned at the stake. There was no public awareness that the "plague of the aged" was a disease until Dr. Alois Alzheimer initially described it in 1907—and even then its intricacies were not understood.

At this very moment, statistics indicate that there are more than 4 million Americans suffering with Alzheimer's. There are over 20 million more people in the role of caregivers and family members who are directly affected by it. If you realize that Alzheimer's is a chronic disease that develops over several decades prior to detection, this estimated 4 million figure swells markedly, as do all related and subsequent statistics. The longer we live, the more likely we are to succumb to it. Fourteen million Americans will be suffering its mental decay thirty-five to forty years from now, and over 70 million family members will be directly affected in the United States alone.

CHANGES IN THE BRAIN

Let us first take a look at the concept of "pathogenicity," the abnormal changes that occur in the brain. "Pathogenicity" or "pathogenesis" refers to the way damage occurs to a brain cell. There are three distinct pathways that lead to this damage. One results from the formation of toxic protein plaques that are abnormal clumps of protein within the brain known as beta-amyloid. These are formed when the normal amyloid protein that is found in the brain undergoes abnormal changes. These toxic protein clumps then induce deformed, twisted, and dead nerve fibers called neurofibrillary tangles and threads. The skeletal remains of these dead nerve cells and fibers are often referred to as "ghosts" and "tombstones" (Grasby 1997); abnormal findings these are the primary features found at autopsy and are the diagnostic hallmark of Alzheimer's disease.

Nerve cell damage, neurofibrillary tangles, and the resultant demise of the neuron, all caused by the abnormal beta-amyloid protein, are present throughout most structures of the brain. The presenting symptoms of this disease are directly related to those areas of the brain that are correspondingly affected. The brain segment subjected to the greatest amount of damage is the hippocampus, the area of learning and memory, and it plays the most crucial role in Alzheimer's. The second most frequently affected area of damage with resultant atrophy (shrinkage of tissue) is in the brain's temporal lobes. Evidence of atrophy in the hippocampus and temporal lobes on scanning modalities (procedures similar to X rays), such as magnetic resonance imaging (MRI) and the positron emission tomography (PET) scan, are diagnostic for Alzheimer's.

Cellular damage prevents electrical impulses from progressing across nerve synapses and continuing along nerve fibers. A synapse is the connection between the end of one nerve cell extension and an adjoining nerve cell. The synapse itself is the minuscule open-cuffed space between the ends of these two structures. The size of this space is minute, measuring one-billionth of an inch. It becomes filled with a liquid known as a neurotransmitter that provides the medium for impulses to travel and traverse the synaptic spaces between nerve endings. Its action is similar to an electrical current traveling along a copper wire and traversing a space to the next wire at a plug-in junction (electric outlet). The plug acts like the neurotransmitter: if it is not inserted into the receptacle, the current is interrupted. Just as a plug conducts our electrical current, the chemical neurotransmitter acetylcholine conducts our nerve impulses. Delays of nerve impulses are due to a decrease in acetylcholine or one of fifty other neurotransmitters. The loss of acetylcholine may be due to chemical or metabolic abnormalities, or from damage or death of the nerve's synaptic connection only, or of the entire nerve cell itself. As a result, the neurotransmitter is unable to conduct electrically charged nerve impulses.

There is significant shrinkage (atrophy) of gray matter in the cortical areas of the brain, and the signal intensity of the brain's white matter, measured by MRI scanning, is significantly increased, as reported by a study at the University of California, San Francisco (Tanabe et al. 1997). Continual shrinkage of the brain's hippocampal segment, as well as the temporal lobes, is a primary diagnostic feature of Alzheimer's disease.

Actual brain volume determines the intellectual reserve, as revealed by studies at the Hyogo Institute in Japan. The larger the brain, the greater the reserve that remains throughout this deteriorating process (Mori et al. 1997).

In a study partly funded by the National Institute on Aging, two theories were proposed. One postulated that dementia does not occur until a significant degree of brain damage has occurred. The other theorizes that dementia is not evident until the brain's reserve drops below a critical level. Interestingly, higher educational levels and larger brain size delay the onset of Alzheimer's (Mortimer 1995).

EARLY MARKERS: THE SENSES

Knowledge of little-known but vital markers of Alzheimer's disease will readily enable us to predict its occurrence, sometimes years before its onset, and these markers can be easily recognized and tested at home.

The course of dementia is now believed to slowly span a period as long as thirty years or more prior to the onset of symptoms, even as early as the fetal stages. We possess greater than 10 billion neurons (nerve cells) at birth, giving our brains significant resiliency. Short-term memory loss is one of the earliest and most prominent symptoms of Alzheimer's, even though long-term memory is still acute during the disease's early stages. Unfortunately, due to its very gradual onset, such memory loss may be inadvertently overlooked, dismissed as part of the normal aging process, or denied by both family and patient. Patients are in fairly good control of mental faculties at the very early stages of dementia and retain decent recognition and thought processes. So they tend to minimize memory loss, attributing it to absent-mindedness or benign forgetfulness. They may realize that the car keys are misplaced, or that they've become lost driving home, or that the checkbook cannot be balanced any longer. They are still cognizant enough to comprehend that they are having difficulties. It is at this early stage of disease, fearing criticism, questioning, or embarrassment, that they cleverly hide these symptoms for as long as their mental faculties permit. They are still too proud to recognize or admit that they are flirting with senility or Alzheimer's, may be in denial themselves, or may dread the loss of independence and role reversal with their children.

We must act as detectives at the earliest suspicion of symptoms. We cannot wait for the barn to burn down before trying to save the horses. Early recognition is the key to treatment and prevention. We will now review some of the very early suggestive symptoms that families have such great difficulty recognizing.

The earliest observable, objective clinical manifestations are short-term memory loss and defects in cognition. The earliest and most diagnostically important cognitive losses, however, involve the senses, and such changes can be detected up to two years before memory loss is observed. Here are five of them:

1. The *sense of smell* is lost approximately two years prior to the onset of most other symptoms. This sensory loss is due to damage or death of a significant number of nerve cells in the olfactory area of the brain, the segment involved with smell. This represents a reliable marker for early diagnosis. Studies conducted at San Diego State University report that odor identification tests have a "correct classification" rate of 83 to 100 percent (Morgan, Norden, and Murphy et al. 1995). Simple tests performed at home can shed early light on the diagnosis. Inability to recognize the aromas of familiar items such as certain foods and prepared dishes, spices, toiletries, and flowers are definite telltale symptoms.

2. *Visual disturbances* occur long before clinical symptoms become apparent. The loss of visual-spatial skills is due to

damage in the parietal-occipital area of the brain Alzheimer's patients, as shown in a study at the National Institutes of Health (NIH). A study using geographic and three-dimensional figures indicates that early difficulties are experienced by Alzheimer's patients with drawing, copying, and following instructions (Fujii et al. 1994).

Another study at the NIH reveals that abnormal brain function due to insufficient blood supply at the visual cortical area mainly in the temporal locations of the brain is involved with visuospatial dysfunction. The PET scan (imaging test) measures lack of blood flow to the involved areas and can accurately measure the brain's metabolism in any given segment (Mentis et al. 1996).

3. *Hearing loss* is extraordinarily high. In a study performed at the University of South Florida, forty-nine of fifty-two Alzheimer's patients had significant loss of hearing (Gold, Lightfoot, and Hnath-Chisholm 1996).

4. *Depression* is also a very early marker. Its average onset is greater than two years prior to the diagnosis of Alzheimer's, and occurs in 50 percent of all Alzheimer's patients, as revealed by studies at the St. Louis University School of Medicine. Symptoms of agitation were studied in this same group, but they did not occur until the first year following diagnosis (Jost and Grossberg 1996). Other symptoms accompanying the dementia, such as paranoia, delusions, and hallucinations, occur in more advanced stages.

Major depression affecting Alzheimer's patients is four times more likely to occur prior to onset of symptoms rather than after the disease becomes evident, in comparison to other dementias (Zubenko et al. 1996). As noted above, this occurs two or more years prior to perceived objective symptoms. Depression is found in half of all Alzheimer's patients, but it also is seen in one-half of all other cases of dementia, regardless of cause.

To summarize, the major differentiating factor is that depression occurs two years prior to the onset of symptoms in Alzheimer's while it does not occur until after the onset of symptoms in other types of dementia.

5. Several cognitive parameters were evaluated in a lengthy and intensive study of a group of 678 convent nuns, prior to demise, and followed by autopsy. One of these was *linguistic ability*. Reviewing the autobiographies of 104 of these nuns, the study revealed that low linguistic ability in their twenties was followed by decreased thought processes later in life and a greater risk of Alzheimer's (Snowdon 1996).

DIAGNOSIS

There are many types of dementias and Alzheimer's is by far the most common, accounting for 70 percent of all known dementias. All dementias are categorized and referred to either as a dementia of the "Alzheimer's type" or as "Alzheimer-related dementias" since the "related dementias" all have different causes from Alzheimer's but have symptoms that may overlap and mimic Alzheimer's. To ensure proper treatment, each must be differentiated from Alzheimer's.

An "Alzheimer-related dementia" such as pernicious anemia, mad cow disease, or a mini-stroke syndrome may occur by itself. Such related dementia may also occur in combination with Alzheimer's, and when this happens, the two together are referred to as mixed dementias. Most often, however, Alzheimer's exists by itself. Pure Alzheimer's accounts for the vast majority of all dementias. Seventy percent of deaths related to dementia are due to pure Alzheimer's disease, as determined at autopsy. Approximately 15 percent of dementia-related deaths are due to the many other causes of related dementias as described in chapter 4, the most frequent of which is vascular disease. The remaining 15 percent of dementias corroborated at autopsy are caused by mixed disease states, which are a combination of Alzheimer's plus one or more of the "Alzheimer-related dementias" (Campion et al. 1996).

Fifty to sixty percent of the diagnoses are totally missed by families, even when they are in constant contact with the patient. Those patients without close family ties, those with families in denial, and those without families at all present with the diagnosis long after the disease process has progressed into its later stages. Diagnosis of Alzheimer's has always been quite difficult to make—even into its intermediate stages—and requires that the physician can reliably exclude the presence of associated dementias as described above.

Only the physician's experience, cognition, and expertise could make the diagnosis in the days prior to neuropsychological testing and laboratory testing and scanning techniques, and only autopsy could provide a definitive diagnosis.

Presently, a definitive diagnosis of Alzheimer's is still not a simple task. It requires a thorough clinical evaluation with blood testing, X rays, neuropsychiatric testing, and scanning procedures by the patient's primary care physician. A second opinion with a neurologist or psychiatrist may be advisable. A 3-D PET scan is the most accurate of all testing modalities, but it is generally not utilized due to its scarcity and huge expense. The newer 3-D SPECT scan is quite helpful, but lower accuracy and greater expense preclude its use in favor of the 3-D MRI scan. Neuropsychological testing is an informative diagnostic tool. Even more difficult than diagnosing a pure Alzheimer's state is the differentiation of an Alzheimer's mixed with related dementias. Diagnostic modalities such as the CAT scan, cerebrospinal fluid testing, and further blood testing may prove essential in differentiating Alzheimer's state from its multiple related dementias since a definitive diagnosis demands exclusion of these related dementias. At times, combined multiple modalities are required to differentiate Alzheimer's from associated dementias, such as the use of a CAT scan along with an MRI at the same time, to evaluate a mixed type of dementia as that described above (Horn et al. 1996).

Although modalities such as the MRI and PET scans are absolutely superb for following the disease's progression, they are no longer really needed once the diagnosis has been made. The patient can then be followed and managed adequately by the physician's expertise and less expensive neuropsychological tests.

Major Breakthroughs in Diagnosis

Throughout the history of the disease, there has not been one specific test diagnostic for Alzheimer's. There are now several exciting major breakthroughs, however, as follows:

Laboratory

AD7C is the newest and most significant test currently available with an accuracy approaching that of autopsy. It measures the elevated level of the neural thread protein found in the brains and spinal fluid of Alzheimer's patients. A spinal tap is required since the test is performed on cerebrospinal fluid. It will soon be marketed as a urine test, however, and when this happens, the ease of securing a specimen and the availability of the test itself can potentially elevate it to the status of a gold standard for early diagnosis of Alzheimer's, assuming it performs as expected.

Scanning Techniques

Scanning techniques (CAT, PET, MRI, and SPECT) have been fair to excellent. Advancements in technology with 3-D (three-dimensional) scanners permit spectacular improvements in diagnosis of Alzheimer's disease.

MRI   The newest 3-D MRI scanner is 95 percent accurate for diagnosis of Alzheimer's.

PET Scan   The newest three-dimensional PET scanning technique is 99 percent specific for diagnosis of Alzheimer's, and is the best test currently available. It measures the flow of blood throughout the brain, as does the SPECT scan, but it is far more accurate. It can measure glucose metabolism in the brain, a feature that enables it to predict Alzheimer's possibly many years in advance of clinical symptoms.

Alzheimer's is liable to be overdiagnosed when proper time and effort are not taken to adequately rule out many related dementias. As a result, the accuracy of the diagnosis is often suspect. Differential diagnosis and earlier recognition of Alzheimer's are now in a state of dynamic change. Although Alzheimer's has been historically a diagnosis of exclusion, this focus is reversing, and the Alzheimer's-related dementias are now becoming the disease states to be excluded. We are on the verge of a quantum leap forward in our ability to differentiate Alzheimer's disease from other disease states, recognize its onset at earlier stages, and intervene much earlier with preventive measures.

COURSE

The clinical hallmarks of Alzheimer's dementia are progression and retrogression.

As the disease progresses through various stages of continuous degenerative processes, the severity of its symptoms is commensurate with the degree of nerve cell damage and death. The particular areas of the brain's involvement and its functions govern the clinical symptoms. For example, frontotemporal dementia occurs as a result of advanced damage in the frontal lobes of the brain. This causes decreased attention and possibly dramatic loss of inhibitions. Another example is that of cellular damage to the olfactory lobes of the brain with subsequent loss of the sense of smell. Cellular death in the hippocampus area of the brain is the most prominent area of Alzheimer involvement and results in the decline and eventual total loss of memory and learning. Nerve cell death in other areas affect hearing, emotions, bladder and bowel control, and other body functions.

Clinically, the disease retrogresses spatially and chronologically, going backward in time, and eventually mimicking the mentality and actions of childhood and infancy. The dementia worsens as more and more brain cells undergo damage and death. Learning wanes. The beautiful memories of a lifetime slowly dissipate into oblivion, lost forever and never again to be enjoyed, never to be recaptured.

The Early Stages

"Short-term memory loss" is the most important perceptive symptom of the early stages of Alzheimer's. Its onset is always subtle and nearly totally overlooked. "Where did I place my hat?" "I can't find my shoes." "You say I missed breakfast?" "Shutting off the electric? But I never saw the bill!" "Are you sure we bought bread yesterday?" "I don't recall the children visiting last week." Occurrences of last week, yesterday, and even five minutes ago are erased or confused. Since other mental faculties at this stage of development are still acute, the patient cleverly hides these very early symptoms. However, the rapidity of change and downward progression varies among patients. If there is intercurrent vascular disease, such as mini-strokes, the course may be far more rapid. As a rule, however, the retrogressing diminution of memory is slow over the course of several years. While memory of recent experiences begins to fade, long-term memory is not yet affected and may still be quite sharp. Names, birth dates, and previous events as far back as childhood are still vivid.

The Intermediate Stages

In the intermediate stages the disease painfully and pathetically progresses through increasing stages of confusion, increased depression, increased memory loss, and mood swings. Typical symptoms include decreased perceptions of time and space, agitation, restlessness, becoming lost, and then the roaming behavior associated with sundowner's syndrome.

The Advanced Stages

Advanced stages of disease are marked by aggressiveness, paranoia, a steady mental deterioration with hallucinations and delusions, refusal to eat, and weight loss. Loss of recognition, loss of the ability to speak, and total incapacitation precede eventual demise.

DEATH AND THE FAMILY

Unfortunately, it is not only the patient who suffers. Alzheimer's dementia impacts the entire family with emotional pain and anguish. Everyone is stricken with sadness, sorrow, and grief as their loved one's health declines. The spiraling downhill passage preceding death inflicts an entire spectrum of emotional pain and suffering upon the devastated families. Some are able to cope quite well; others are severely traumatized and totally shattered.

Because family members may not fully understand what is happening or how to respond, they may overindulge the patient with their expressions of love and behave as if in denial. They consciously (knowingly) or subconsciously (unknowingly) avoid facing reality. Therefore, avoidance, along with denial, are normal psychological and self-protective responses used by family members.

Guilt surfaces in the family during the intermediate stage, if not earlier, and crests prior to the demise of the loved one. Many family members become engulfed with fear of genetic inheritance. Two-thirds of caregivers react with anger, and over 50 percent of them experience reactive depression. Most become frustrated and can't cope well with stress, and their own immune systems suffer as their anxieties and frustrations mount.

Life expectancy of Alzheimer's patients can range between two and twenty years after the diagnosis is made, but survival is generally six to eight years. Some authorities claim that senility ushers in a ten- to twenty-year life expectancy, while Alzheimer's forecasts a three- to five-year life expectancy following diagnosis. Most authorities, however, agree that the full course of the disease slowly spans thirty or more years. According to Dr. R. L. Blaylock of Jackson, Mississippi, the disease process may even start as early as the fetal stage, secondary to oxygen deprivation, glucose deprivation, vitamin deficiencies in the brain, amino acid imbalances, or other metabolic abnormalities, all of which create cellular damage. (These are explained in detail under "Causes" in chapter 6.) Death may result due to a lifetime of slowly recurring and intermittent insults to brain tissues. Appropriate early intervention can prevent many, if not most, of these changes (Blaylock 1996).

A study done at the Mayo Clinic comparing causes of deaths of all patients in the Alzheimer's group versus nondemented patients yielded an important piece of information. The control group expired mostly from cardiovascular disease and cancer. The Alzheimer's group, on the other hand, died more often from bronchitis and pneumonia (Beard 1996). Pneumonia is the greatest immediate cause of death in Alzheimer's patients. A depressed immune system, frequent aspiration of food and liquid due to poorer swallowing functions, muscle weakness that decreases the strength of coughing, and increased recumbency all enable pneumonia to take its deadly toll.

When death occurs, it is often said that it comes as mercy to the patient and a sad relief to the caregiver.

COSTS

Business losses in the United States from absenteeism and decreased productivity of spouses, sons, or daughters who must act as caregivers to ailing loved ones at home is far in excess of $30 billion per year, and even that is a gross underestimate. The combined expenses of research, diagnosis, medication, caregiving, treatment, and institutionalization for Alzheimer's disease is well in excess of $100 billion per year—greater than the total operating budgets of many countries around the world.

It is estimated that just slowing down the progression of the disease will save as much as $50 billion per year (Mecks 1997). Enormous leaps in technology have enabled us to significantly reduce the costs of diagnosis. With earlier diagnosis, better treatments, and elements of prevention now attainable, we will see fewer illnesses and, with that, a decreased need for physician visits, hospitalizations, and long-term care facilities, thus resulting in markedly reduced expense.

WHAT ARE MY CHANCES OF GETTING ALZHEIMER'S?

Alzheimer's is a disease that primarily affects those in their late sixties and seventies, with the majority of cases commonly occurring past age sixty-five. However, it can be seen as early as the thirties and forties, but its occurrence at earlier ages indicates definite genetic mutations. Approximately 10 percent of the population will develop Alzheimer's before age sixty-five.

With a totally negative family history, the risk of developing Alzheimer's is 15 percent over the span of your lifetime (de la Torre 1996). That's 1.5 out of every 10 people, but if you think that's bad, just wait! If one of your first-degree relatives has Alzheimer's, your risk of developing it increases to 39 percent, or roughly four chances in ten (Lautenschlager et al. 1996). And if both of your parents have or have had the disease, your risk of developing it is 54 percent before age eighty (Lautenschlager et al. 1996). What is even more frightening, irrespective of whether one or both parents did or did not have the disease, is that approximately 50 percent of the total population who live past age eighty-five will develop Alzheimer's. However, if it's any consolation, the risk and incidence do decrease again after the age of ninety (Lautenschlager et al. 1996).

There appears to be a definite gender bias in Alzheimer's:

- Women have a twofold risk versus men of developing late-onset Alzheimer's, and this is associated with a genetic inheritance (Payami et al. 1996).
- Women have a greater tendency to develop language difficulties
- Women have a greater tendency to develop psychiatric problems (Lautenschlager et al. 1996) while progressing on a downward spiral
- The speed of progression of the disease leading to dementia and death is significantly faster in selected male groups than in females (Farrer et al. 1995).

Regardless of gender, diabetics have less risk for developing Alzheimer's because high glucose levels appear to protect against its development. The average risk for a person with a negative family background developing the disease is 15 percent, and the diabetic risk is 8.8 percent, or approximately one-half (Itagaki et al. 1996).

Unfortunately, the opposite holds true with people who have low blood sugar since the risk associated with hypoglycemia is nearly double. This group not only includes genetically oriented hypoglycemia but possibly also those persons with poor eating habits, recurrent crash diets, starvation diets, unquestionably inadequate nutrition, and certain metabolic disorders. A temporary lack of sugar has the potential to adversely affect the metabolism of brain cells, interfere with their energy production, and result in cellular death. With 10 billion neurons in the brain at birth, there are no immediate discernible effects. With prolonged abuse and the addition of other causative factors, however, the chances increase for Alzheimer's to eventually manifest itself.

A race and ethnic variation has also been found. In a comparison study between African-Americans, Hispanics, and whites, those who are genetically predisposed to Alzheimer's show no statistical variation between race or ethnicity. In those subjects possessing no genetic predisposition, African-Americans have a risk four times greater than that of whites, and Hispanics evince a 2.5 times greater risk than whites (Ming-Xin et al. 1998).

Genetic Links

The younger someone develops Alzheimer's, the more likely the causative factor is an inherited gene (Masters et al. 1997). It is estimated that up to 20 percent of all Alzheimer's cases are related to genetic inheritance.

Individuals carrying a specific inherited mutated gene named apolipoprotein E 4 (APOE 4) comprise 30 percent of the U.S. population. Only 10 percent of these carriers will develop Alzheimer's, and APOE 4 does not affect its rate of progression. Although it may predispose the patient to the disease, it does not appear to accelerate the patient's decline. The other 90 percent of carriers do not develop Alzheimer's, but they may pass on this abnormal gene (mutation) to their offspring.

Late-onset disease is both familial and sporadic. Fifteen percent of familial cases are now traced to a newly discovered gene on chromosome #12.

MAJOR BREAKTHROUGHS IN TREATMENT

Prevention of Alzheimer's dementia was previously synonymous with "wishful thinking" because we had very little to offer aside from superb caregiving. Two drugs were approved by the Food and Drug Administration (FDA) and marketed for the treatment of Alzheimer's: tacrine (Cognex) and donepezil (Aricept). Although helpful, they offer no prevention. Selegiline, a drug used in the treatment of Parkinson's disease, was found to be far superior in the long term because it possesses antioxidant and other properties, combinations that afford protection against the progression of Alzheimer's. Further research reveals that a number of other prescription and nonprescription agents such as estrogen, vitamin E, ibuprofen, nicotine, Tagamet, and coenzyme Q10, surprisingly, are significantly effective against Alzheimer's disease. Further independent research reveals that Alzheimer patients are deficient in thiamine (vitamin B_1) and the amino acid tyrosine.

CHAPTER 3

Symptoms

The most frequently asked questions about Alzheimer's are: "How can I tell?" "What are the symptoms?" "What do I look for?" "How do I know?" "What can I do?" "What can I expect?" "Where can I get information?" "Why didn't someone tell me?" "How will the course of the disease progress?"

THE SYMPTOMS OF ALZHEIMER'S

Numerous symptoms follow a set course of decline. Although there may be a wide spectrum of demented actions and not every patient will exhibit every symptom, a downhill regression follows a general pattern of mental regression and physical decline. Early markers of an evolving disease process involve the senses of smell, hearing, and vision, along with pre-dementia depression. The earlier these initial symptoms are recognized, the greater the chances are to slow and prevent the progression of dementia. Although some of these have been previously mentioned, they bear repeating here.

Short-Term Memory Loss

Short-term memory loss is usually the first perceived and most critical objective symptom. It can present itself very subtly. Initially, the patient is aware of the errors and cleverly hides them.

Eventually, though, the short-term memory loss becomes increasingly evident to family and friends, and other newly surfacing symptoms raise the levels of suspicion that a dementia is evolving. Questions such as "Who stole the car keys?" "What's your name again?" "Which car is ours?" "Why is the ice cream in the cupboard and who put it there?" and "How do you unlock the microwave oven?" are difficult to ignore.

Confusion, Disorientation, and Wandering

Confusion follows closely on the heels of memory loss, and they coalesce. Simple tasks and procedures become increasingly difficult. A person places a shoe on one foot and a sneaker on the other, then thinks, "Fine, but how do I tie them?" Operation of the microwave becomes daunting: "Are you sure I warmed the frying pan in the microwave oven?" Food preparation is a challenge: "Do I remove the head from that fish or mix it in the salad?" Simple tasks and procedures become difficult. Finding the route home from the store, balancing the bank statement, writing simple checks, and coordinating clothes become more and more difficult and confusing. Mixing up the names and faces of children and grandchildren is a common occurrence.

Disorientation is a prominent feature. The patient loses contact with time and space. Driving skills are still maintained early in the course of the disease. Gradually, due to spatial disorientation and confusion, difficulties occur in arriving at the intended destination and then returning home. However, the patient is unaware of the loss of these skills, and this creates a greater burden on the caregiver, who must decide when to restrict driving. Typically, the patient reacts with greater depression, agitation, and possibly anger when faced with relinquishing that last threshold of independence. Obviously, caution and safety are the primary concerns when it becomes necessary to confiscate the car keys; the caregiver cannot permit the first auto mishap.

Eventually, spatial disorientation will occur even walking to and from the house. The patient who walks away from home and forgets where home is, and how to return, is referred to as a "wanderer" or a "walker," and caregiving for that person mandates tight home security. Wandering will surface in the intermediate stage and worsen in the advanced stage. In time the patient may become lost even inside the home, having difficulty distinguishing the route between the bathroom and the bedroom or kitchen.

Personal Care

Personal care begins to slide. The daily bath becomes a once- or twice-a-week event. Hair is rarely brushed, much less washed. Dressing without assistance in the morning can yield some interesting results: a scanty slip in the depths of winter, boxer shorts or a shirt and nothing else, four or five layers of mismatched clothing in midsummer, legs inside shirtsleeves, or shoes on the wrong foot. Eventually, personal care ebbs entirely, and the caregiver steps in to help the patient with daily hygiene. The caregiver's well-intentioned efforts may first be met with resistance, then verbal abuse, and even aggressiveness and combativeness, often to significant levels.

Although symptoms can vary widely, regression follows a similar course with all Alzheimer patients. To ease your own emotional trauma somewhat, be prepared for your patient or loved one to serially spiral downward through the stages of Alzheimer's dementia. Great patience and perseverance are required by the caregiver to gain trust and cooperation from the patient who is going through the stages of Alzheimer's.

Mood Swings

Mood swings that vary from day to day, even from moment to moment, mark the intermediate stages. Patients may be happy and singing aloud one moment, then crying the next without any apparent reason. They may have wild arguments with the TV set, believing that the performers are addressing them directly, or they may have delusional conversations with a pillow, an article of furniture, a clothes tree, or any inanimate object. Instructions or questions may be met by refusal to answer, an angry response, or a possible storm of verbal and physical abuse.

Restlessness is characteristic, and pacing floors, opening and closing of hallway or cabinet doors, being unable to relax, and constantly mumbling nonsensical and disjointed words are typical symptoms of the intermediate period of dementia.

The Sundowner's Syndrome

It is during this stage of disease progression that the sundowner's syndrome blossoms. This constellation of behaviors is a hallmark of Alzheimer's disease. Toward dusk, just before the sun goes down, the decrease in light intensity has an adverse effect on the brain. The patient becomes even more hyperactive and may pace the floor throughout the night and early morning hours, keeping the entire household awake. This is due, in part, to a deficiency of melatonin, a hormone-like substance that controls the day/night activity of the brain known as circadian rhythms. Oral supplementation of melatonin and some herbal supplements may help alleviate symptoms. Curiously, this hyperactivity and perpetual motion can stop abruptly, and patients may stand and stare into nothingness as if in a catatonic stupor. The converse is equally true, whereby patients are totally withdrawn and would spend twenty to twenty-four hours lying in bed if permitted to do so. These behavior patterns may recur interchangeably and unpredictably without rhyme or reason. They may be interlaced with any one of countless behavioral changes at any given time.

Throughout the early and intermediate stages, patients will experience good and bad days. During good days, early in the course of disease, families may be deluded into thinking that the diagnosis has been in error because their loved one appears to improve, but eventually the good days become less frequent, then sporadic, and later they are reduced to fleeting moments only.

Eating Habits and Weight Loss

Eating habits become increasingly erratic. Patients require greater periods of time to eat meals and may (at times) just sit and refuse to eat. Toward the end of the early stages, patients become confused about the use of silverware, with attempts to cut with a spoon and stir with a fork or knife. By the late intermediate stages, they often become confused about chewing. It is not unusual to observe someone sitting with a mouth half-filled for as long as an hour if not encouraged to chew. Taking medications can be problematic:

patients may be observed placing pills or capsules into their beverages and either stirring them, spooning them, or playing with them instead of taking them properly. Pouring a beverage over a plate of food will happen instead of drinking it. Like a child or infant just learning to eat, the patient may sit playing with food or may stop drinking and eating altogether. Intermittent assisted feeding is required in the intermediate stage and becomes a routine necessity late in the course of the disease.

Patients actually do much better without silverware. When the meal is planned to incorporate the use of finger foods, patients eat better and achieve greater nourishment, and less burden is placed upon the caregiver. Liquid food supplements such as Ensure, Nutramigen, and Sustacal should be included into the diet to ensure continued nutrition. These supplements are readily available in pharmacies and grocery stores.

There is slow but progressive weight loss throughout the course of the disease. Total body weight can drop below 100 pounds, depending on height and bone structure. At the final stage of disease, prior to death, weight can plummet into the 70- to 80-pound range. As nutrition suffers, the strength of the immune system slowly wanes and infections become increasingly common. As previously noted, pneumonia generally becomes the great equalizer.

In the very late or terminal stages, a feeding tube introduced into the stomach through the abdominal wall may eventually be the only way to provide nourishment, particularly when the patient reaches a semivegetative state. Although the procedure is not complicated for a physician, permission for a feeding tube is an extremely difficult decision for a family to grant. It is grievous to see a loved one in a semivegetative state. Can we even think of such a state as a "quality of life" issue? Should every effort be made to prolong life? Should heroics be employed against intercurrent life-threatening emergencies? Should most measures be withheld and allow Providence to take its course? These are monumental and extremely difficult decisions to make, and it is at this level that depression and guilt experienced by family members reach their zeniths.

Depression

Depression is experienced by 50 percent of all Alzheimer's patients and is characterized by withdrawal, melancholy, apathy, and crying. Although depression is also found in fully half of Alzheimer's-related dementias, the timing of its onset is unique in Alzheimer's, separating it from all other dementias. It is referred to as pre-dementia depression because it occurs up to two years or more before the onset of Alzheimer's symptoms, which red-flags it as a marker for this dementia. In non-Alzheimer's-related diseases, the depression occurs well after the onset of dementia itself.

Treatment for depression is relatively straightforward because we have several classes of effective prescription medications available today, such as the tricyclics, the dopamine receptor agonists (helpers), and the type known as serotonin reuptake inhibitors. Some of he most popular antidepressants are Prozac, Paxil, and Effexor.

St. John's wort, a nonprescription herbal medicine of increasing popularity, is an inexpensive and very effective antidepressant, devoid of nearly all side effects. It is used worldwide, especially in Europe, and is gaining rapid acceptance in the United States with greater than a 2,000 percent increase in usage over the past year. St. John's wort is reputed to be as effective as Prozac and acts in a similar manner with far fewer side effects.

Agitation

Agitation is observed throughout all stages of Alzheimer's. In the early stages of dementia it is mild and initially may not differ clinically from frustration. It becomes more obvious when patients are seen to be mentally disturbed and upset, when they may display quick tempers or respond with unkind words. At first, patients will appear disturbed about entirely inconsequential occurrences such as minor lapses of memory associated with normal daily activities and routines. They exhibit their feelings verbally or by intense facial and body expressions. Difficulty relaxing or going to sleep further worsens their emotional state as patients regress and become more and more difficult to manage. When anger and hostility surface, the caregiver's patience can be sorely tested.

Although many prescription medications can control these symptoms including anxiolytics (tranquilizers), sedatives, and hypnotics (sleeping medications), they all can have side effects. Of interest are a few safe, mild, and effective herbal products that provide relaxation and sleep such as valerian root, passionflower, and kava, readily available at pharmacies and health food stores. At lower doses, they act as anxiolytics during the day; at higher doses, they act as sedatives or hypnotics at night.

Aggression

Aggression soon accompanies agitation as the intermediate stage evolves, and it progresses in a crescendo fashion durning the late stages. Aggression can manifest itself in many ways. Patients may become verbally abusive and may use street vocabulary never before uttered. They may be physically abusive, hitting or pushing family members or strangers without warning or provocation. These actions are most often directed against the caregiver. Alzheimer's victims literally do strike or bite the hand that feeds them.

That caregiving is difficult is a vast understatement, but there are many effective strategies to offset such aggression:

- Try to prevent any known precipitating causes of mental or emotional stress.
- If aggressive behavior has already begun, act immediately to separate the stimulus from the patient.
- Quickly refocus disturbing thought processes: create non-provocative alternative outlets.
- Encourage repetitive activities since these relieve stress on the patient.
- Avoid sudden, stressful change of environment in later stages.
- Because sunlight is calming, open all blinds, and try to give access to a bright environment.
- Be gentle, reassuring, and patient.
- Never express anger in voice, attitude, or actions since these precipitate similar reactions from the patient.

To summarize: avoidance of stress, diversion, shift of the patient's thought processes, distractions from present agitation and frustration, avoidance of environmental change, and copious sunlight are valid interventions. We must always remember that Alzheimer's patients are totally unaware of their actions and certainly not responsible for them since they have lost considerable brain tissue, memory, and the ability to reason. Alzheimer's is an illness, and its victims must be treated with compassion.

Paranoia

Paranoia, an abnormal thought process marked by irrational thinking, can occur with or without Alzheimer's or other related dementias: it can present by itself with no other disease state. Paranoia is a state of mind that causes its victim to become distrustful and suspicious of others. These patients harbor the conviction that people are plotting against them or that the police, FBI, KGB, detectives, or invaders from outer space are following them. Such patients can be so convincing as they describe their adversaries or pursuers that even their therapists may be thrown off guard and initially swayed by them. Alzheimer's patients will misinterpret other people's whispers, talk, or laughter, and think that it is directed toward them. They react abruptly, make accusations, falsify or fabricate stories, and even fantasize escape routes or go into hiding. Money is a major concern in paranoia of Alzheimer's dementia. Because patients constantly suspect that others are stealing from them, they hide their money, bankbooks, and valuables. As the paranoia progresses, things get worse, and Alzheimer's patients begin to hoard and hide other items: clothing, jewelry, old shoes, kitchen utensils, and anything that's not nailed down and that they can carry. These items are later found in odd places such as under the bed, in drawers, in cabinets and storage areas, in the shower, in suitcases, under the sink, and just about anywhere that is accessible to them.

Their ideations become fixated to such a degree that they can appear delusional. Thus, their paranoia can actually coexist with delusions.

Delusions

Delusions are completely false ideations and unshakable beliefs that are firmly fixed in one's mind, and occur in more than 40 percent of all Alzheimer's patients. For example, they may believe that they are visiting with dead relatives and ask repeatedly if anyone else has seen these deceased relatives today, totally unaware that they are, in fact, dead. They are so convinced of their beliefs that you should not try to dissuade them unless you are prepared to face a scornful confrontation. Lengthy and emotionally charged conversations with stuffed toys, pillows, or imagined visitors are common. Angry or aggressive conversations may be held with the television, and, depending upon the context of the program, a patient may throw food or drink at the TV in a fit of anger. Interestingly, programs with young children appear to have a calming effect while news channels and violent programs appear to provoke outbursts. Some patients will regress into childlike behavior; they may carry stuffed toys or dolls and nurture them as one would care for an infant or a young child by giving them food and drinks.

The FDA has approved the use of Risperdal, a psychotherapeutic drug, for the treatment of delusions, agitation, emotional outbursts, and harsh vocalizations. It is quite effective in ameliorating many of these symptoms, and it may actually be more helpful for the caregiver because it calms the patient.

Hallucinations

Hallucinations are abnormal audiovisual sensory encounters that aren't based on reality. No one but the patient sees or hears them. Typical hallucinatory experiences include seeing spiders or bugs crawling over everything—on the walls, across the ceiling, over bedclothes and furniture. Nonexistent people are seen hiding in bushes. Children, workmen, or groups of people may be perceived as being in the room, when, in fact, no one else is present. Patients may even prepare meals for these imaginary guests and then may have lengthy conversations with them.

Hallucinations are not restricted to Alzheimer's or other dementias. They are seen in nondemented patients; in people who suffer from psychoses (loss of contact with reality) such as schizophrenia, in people who suffer from neuroses (nervous patients); and in otherwise normal people.

Fortunately, there are a number of strategies to treat these abnormal states of mind. Prescription drugs can measurably calm or ameliorate these conditions. Psychiatrists and psychologists are readily available and quite capable of providing help. However, caregiver assistance is paramount since they are the people closest to, and the most concerned about, the patient. Here is a list of do's and don'ts for caregivers:

- Recognize that what is an abnormality to us seems totally real to the patient.
- Never disagree or try to convince the patient that what he or she sees or hears does not exist.
- Never ridicule, reproach, or mock the patient's beliefs because they are a very serious matter to him or her.
- Talk to their stuffed toys or imaginary visitors with them to provide reassurance and confirmation of their beliefs.
- Become a source of greater security for the patient.

It may not always be the easiest of chores, but it will minimize much of the patients' frustration, anger, agitation, and aggressiveness, and it will lessen the strain placed upon the caregivers. When the caregiver is the patient's own child, a stressful and often painful role reversal occurs in which the caregiver (the child who has reached adulthood) must assume the role of surrogate parent for his or her own parent (whose mind has regressed to that of childhood). Even the grandchildren become participants in such role reversals.

Hallucinations, delusions, and paranoia may overlap one another, or they may all coexist. With deepening regression, however, these mental difficulties slowly subside as that stage of dementia is reached where there is not even enough viable brain tissue remaining to support these abnormal thought processes.

Incontinence

Incontinence of urine is a symptom of late-stage disease. By this stage of regression, the more important mental faculties are lost. Barring any associated physical disorder (such as a dropped uterus in a woman or prostate disease in a man, or disease of the urethra, bladder, or kidney), urinary incontinence (loss of ability to hold urine) may be the result of neuronal brain cell damage and death. Bowel incontinence (loss of control) may soon follow. Although end-stage disease may usher in incontinence of urine or bowel, death generally occurs before these symptoms surface.

Long-term care facilities are often inadequately staffed to provide optimum frequency of diaper changes and proper skin care, and many Alzheimer's patients suffer from skin irritation, pressure sores, local infections, and eventually skin breakdown known as "decubitus ulcers." It is less damaging for the skin and easier for the attendants if the patients have indwelling catheters inserted, but even this procedure has drawbacks because, even with meticulous care, it can cause recurring urethral and bladder infections. The greatest risk is that infection may spread retrograde (upward through the ureters) into the kidney or, worse, into the bloodstream, causing generalized infection known as bacteremia or septicemia. If, as often happens, this blood-borne infection spreads to the brain, it creates a toxic encephalopathy (an inflammation and swelling of brain tissue) resulting in acute inflammatory dementia and psychosis (mental confusion). The patient will then lose further contact with reality and mimic any of the mental symptoms seen in dementia, further worsening the preexisting symptoms of Alzheimer's.

Speech Loss

The mild speech difficulties in the early stages of disease are irritating and frustrating. Patients who maintain their mental faculties may fully realize their intended thoughts but are unable to express them adequately. Family members and caregivers must be patient and understanding.

The intermediate stage is ushered in by slowly advancing difficulties with speech. Sentences and thoughts become disjointed and there is inability to focus and stay with one subject. Verbalizing grows increasingly worse to the point where dysphasia (difficulty speaking) ensues and conversation and speech are no longer coherent.

In advanced stages of disease, *aphasia* (inability to speak more than a few words or sounds) sets in, and nonsensical phrases or words are the maximum capability.

Total Incapacitation and Death

The final stage of Alzheimer's disease is marked by total incapacitation. This represents the last of the body's failing faculties prior to demise. The symptom complex and timetable vary from patient to patient but will continue to exhibit a pattern of physical and mental regression. Patients may still be ambulatory when a fatal pneumonia or intercurrent malady such as a stroke, heart attack, or cancer takes its toll. Most, however, are wheelchair bound at the time of demise.

Once the disease becomes entrenched it can no longer be prevented, and it will eventually run its full course. Death can come at any age or any stage of dementia.

CHAPTER 4

Alzheimer's-Related Dementias

The diagnosis of Alzheimer's has always been a complex, difficult, and imprecise science. Historically, it has either been ruled in or ruled out based upon the exclusion of other physical and mental symptoms, and other disease states, while the patient was alive. Positive identification based on specific changes in the brain could only be verified by autopsy following the patient's death. Now, however, tremendous strides in new technologies for laboratory testing and monumental innovations with scanning procedures have improved our diagnostic abilities. Alzheimer's dementia can be much more easily and accurately separated from the many other related dementias and diseases that clinically overlap it.

To fully understand the challenge of an accurate diagnosis, it is important to know that there are many related dementias that may exist separately from Alzheimer's-type dementia. There are also mixed dementias that are a combination of Alzheimer's coexisting with one or more of its related dementias. It is this combination of mixed dementias that complicates matters and makes the accurate diagnosis of Alzheimer's a much more difficult task.

Of significant importance, patients who exhibit severe isolated memory loss without any other noticeable cognitive loss must be closely monitored and evaluated since the chances are quite high that they will develop dementia (Bowen et al. 1997). Early diagnosis and treatment are crucial at this juncture; they can be lifesaving.

DEMENTIA

Dementia is defined as "suffering with memory loss plus a minimum of one other cognitive impairment" (Bowen et al. 1997). Some examples of decline in cognition are decreased judgment, time or spatial deterioration, reduction in language skills, behavioral changes, loss of smell, and diminished hearing (Exhibit 4.1.).

While these acquired disease states are probably not reversible, some of them, such as epilepsy, are treatable and potentially controllable. Others, such as Lou Gehrig's and Pick's disease, are genetic and definitely not reversible.

Vascular Dementia

Vascular dementia is the most common of the Alzheimer "related dementias" (Rosler et al. 1996), and it can take many different paths. If it is caused by a very slow development of atherosclerosis over many years' duration during which time the blood supply to the brain is slowly decreased, it can evolve with a prolonged onset, similar to Alzheimer's. The brain suffers cell damage and cell death due to oxygen and sugar deprivation.

This type of dementia can evolve in a stepwise fashion following repeated TIAs (transient ischemic attacks) that are really mini-stroke syndromes. Usually, the patient is totally unaware that a TIA has even occurred. There may be varying transitory symptoms such as light-headedness, dizziness, visual disturbance, headache, or mild tingling of the extremities. More profound easily recognizable, temporary symptoms are slurred speech, drooping face, extremity or facial tingling, fainting, or limb weakness. Dementia may surface after repeated episodes of these mini-strokes, but this depends completely upon which intracranial (brain) arteries are involved, to what extent, whether caused by blockage or hemorrhage, and the number of episodes that occur.

Memory is much more severely impaired in early Alzheimer's than it is in vascular dementia of prolonged onset. As the depths of dementia progress, the vascular type speeds up its development and catches up with Alzheimer's at the stage of moderate impairment (Bowler et al. 1997).

The dementia can present with sudden paralyzing onset following an acute cerebrovascular accident (CVA), also called a major stroke. The severity of damage depends upon which artery and corresponding segment of the brain are involved. There are over 730,000 strokes per year, including both initial and recurrent episodes.

Vascular dementias are not reversible once significant cell death occurs to the brain. During an acute CVA (stroke) due to blockage of a major blood vessel, however, a clot-dissolving medicine that is used for treatment of heart attacks, such as streptokinase or TPA, can be injected and can prevent severe and irreversible damage from occurring if administered in time. Thus, the onset of a potential post-stroke dementia can be prevented. Even newer medicines are now providing some improvement after damage has occurred. Oral blood thinners are now in common use.

Depression

Although depression is not a true "related dementia," it must be discussed along with Alzheimer's and its related dementias because of its prevalence and intregal relationship. It is seen in 50

Exhibit 4.1   Related Dementias

The following are Alzheimer's-related dementias, and they comprise 15 percent of all non-Alzheimer dementias. Vascular diseases (strokes) are the most common and the most important of this group.

PROBABLY NOT REVERSIBLE: ACQUIRED AND GENETIC

Vascular Diseases

     Atherosclerosis (hardening of the arteries) affecting the brain
     Transient ischemic attacks (TIAs); mini-stroke syndromes; strokes (CVAs)

Alcoholism

     Korsakoff's syndrome
     Organic brain syndrome

Metabolic

     Dementia of pernicious anemia (Vitamin B_{12} deficiency)

Infectious

     Chronic virus: Creutzfeldt-Jakob (mad cow disease)

     AIDS
     Neurosyphilis
     Herpes zoster (shingles) dementia

Intracranial Mass

     Cancer

Neurologic

     Progressive supranuclear palsy
     Frontotemporal dementia (potential loss of all inhibitions)
     Pick's disease
     Parkinson's disease
     Amytrophic lateral sclerosis (Lou Gehrig's disease)
     Epilepsy

Exhibit 4.1 Related Dementias, *continued*

PROBABLY REVERSIBLE: ACQUIRED

Encephalopathy (brain swelling)

> Acute infection: bacterial, viral
> Trauma
> Tumor
> Post-stroke
> Renal (kidney) disease
> Hepatic (liver) disease

Intracranial mass

> Tumor
> Hydrocephalus

Infectious

> Recurring Virus: Herpes Simplex Meningitis (if no genetic links)
> Fungal Infections
> Encephalitis

Endocrine: hypothyroid (underactive)

Drug toxicity: patent medicine; prescription drugs; illicit drugs

Psychiatric

> Depression

> Schizophrenia

> Other psychoses

Metabolic

Folic acid: folate anemia

> Electrolyte/mineral imbalance

> Hypoglycemia (low blood sugar)

> Thiamine Deficiencies (vitamin B_1)

> Tyrosine (amino acid) deficiency

> Tryptophan deficiency

> Vitamin B_3 (niacin) deficiency

> Pellagra

percent of all dementias. Since it is often overlooked and its significance minimized, it is often not addressed or treated properly. Depression may occur as a distinct entity. Of all depressions, half are considered severe and thus classified as major depression. The other half are less striking and classified as minor depression. The most severe are those culminating in suicide, and the mildest are those that show minimal or negligible symptoms even though they may exist in a chronic state for years.

Major depression is prevalent in many dementias and is more frequent and more severe with vascular dementia than in those patients suffering with Alzheimer's (Ballard et al. 1996). It surfaces in vascular disease well after onset of the dementia, in contrast to the depression of Alzheimer's, which is less severe but whose onset precedes the dementia by as long as two years. The pre-dementia depression of Alzheimer's is a marker (an early warning sign). Dementia-related depression is treatable, but the response to treatment is not always what is hoped for.

Alzheimer's is the primary suspect when depression without a discernible cause presents by itself during a person's sixties and seventies. It compounds an already difficult diagnosis when it presents in mixed dementias; it is often hard enough to determine which dementias are present, let alone which one is responsible for the depression.

It is known that depression is often triggered by a chemical imbalance in the brain, most frequently due to a deficiency of serotonin, a particular neurotransmitter. To prolong serotonin's neurotransmitter action at the nerve synapse (connector between nerves), the return (reuptake) of this chemical from the synaptic space back into the nerve cell must be delayed (inhibited). Of the three major classes of antidepressants in use today, the most frequently prescribed are serotonin reuptake inhibitors such as Prozac, Zoloft, Effexor, and Paxil, all of which are effective and relatively safe for these patients (Borne 1994).

St. John's wort is an herbal medicinal that has been used worldwide for the treatment of depression for centuries and is allegedly as effective as Prozac without the side effects. It inhibits the reuptake of serotonin by 50 percent, thus prolonging its action and allowing this neurotransmitter to prevent depression and function effectively in the body.

A recent discovery has hypothesized that a deficiency of omega-3 oil, and one of its components in particular, DHA (docosahexaenoic acid), an essential polyunsaturated fatty acid, may be responsible for depression. This essential fatty acid is an integral component of the cell walls found in nerve synapses. It is also abundant in the walls of red blood cells, and these cell membranes are used to measure the amount of this fatty acid in the body. Omega-3 is depleted in depression, and the lower its level drops, the worse the depression (Edwards et al. 1998). Taking a daily supplement of omega-3, such as a tablespoon of flaxseed oil, may be beneficial in the treatment of depression.

Hypothyroidism

Hypothyroidism, the result of an underactive thyroid gland, is very common and increases in incidence with aging. The thyroid is the master gland of the body because it affects every organ system. When it is sluggish, all the body's organ systems also slow down, and any single or multiple group of body systems may exhibit clinical symptoms predicated upon the degree of deficiency in thyroid hormone production.

In a mild case of an underactive thyroid, there may be no

symptoms. As the disease progresses, the many organ systems of the body begin to show signs of slowing down as shown in Exhibit 4.2.

If severe hypothyroidism is left untreated, congestive heart failure and death can occur. All of the symptoms of thyroid deficiency—including dementia—are totally reversible with oral thyroid hormone replacement.

Vitamin B_{12} and Folate Deficiency

B_{12} deficiency is eventually a fatal disease if left untreated, as was the case prior to discovery and replacement of this most essential vitamin. It often occurs in conjunction with folic acid deficiencies. Both are a substantial problem in our elderly population.

Many studies show that serum vitamin B_{12} levels are significantly lower in older people, and that this deficiency is more frequent in Alzheimer's patients than in normal counterparts (Cole and Prchal 1984; Joosten et al. 1997).

When there is a serious deficiency of vitamin B_{12} pernicious anemia can occur. Late-stage symptoms can mimic Alzheimer's dementia. Vitamin B_{12} supplementation will reverse the vitamin deficiency and symptoms of pernicious anemia, but unfortunately dementia due to vitamin B_{12} deficiency cannot be reversed. Although low B_{12} levels are recognized as a definite problem in the elderly and pernicious anemia is common, fortunately the incidence of B_{12} dementia is uncommon. If dementia is observed in a patient with confirmed pernicious anemia, Alzheimer's is more likely the real culprit (Teunisse et al. 1996). If symptoms of pernicious anemia are suspected, a simple blood test may be sufficient to make the diagnosis, or a more accurate

---

Exhibit 4.2 Clinical Symptoms of Hypothyroidism

Organ systems of the body show signs of slowing down:

Ten percent of depressed patients have borderline hypothyroidism

Skin becomes dry

Hair shafts are thicker

Bowel becomes sluggish

Urine may flow with less frequency and volume

Menstrual flow slows, and periods may become irregular and sometimes scant

There may be difficulty becoming pregnant

Muscle strength may wane

Weight gain is so common that thyroid function tests are routine when evaluating obesity

Cholesterol levels increase

Atherogenic process (hardening of the arteries) accelerates

Intolerance to cold occurs

Tiredness is pronounced

In the more serious cases, prominent symptoms may include:

Mental confusion

Lassitude

Garbled speech secondary to a thickened tongue

Shortness of breath

Telltale signs may include:

Slowing of the heart rate

Puffy face

Bagginess under the eyes

Very dry, scaly, flaking skin

Swelling of the lower legs and feet

Dementia (can mimic Alzheimer's)

---

test that measures methylmalonic acid (a B_{12} metabolite) will provide the answer.

When there is a folic acid deficiency, folic acid anemia occurs; changes in the blood resemble those of pernicious anemia. It is also fully reversible with supplementation. Folate and B_{12} deficiencies frequently accompany one another. Folic acid is important nutritionally for prevention of diseases of the nervous system and is now widely prescribed for pregnant women to prevent spina bifida, a birth defect involving the neural (spinal) cord. B_{12} and folate replacement are strongly recommended for Alzheimer's.

Frontotemporal Dementia

Frontotemporal dementia is an uncommon neurodegenerative disease. As the name implies, the pathology is located in the temples and front part of the brain. Its initial clinical attribute is the loss of attention. It can be very difficult, if not nearly impossible, to clinically differentiate from Alzheimer's (Mendez et al. 1996).

However, clinical symptoms indicate some variation from Alzheimer's and are limited to a narrower range of abnormalities than the wide spectrum seen in Alzheimer's. The set of behavioral problems that mark this dementia involves the total disintegration of inhibitions. The more posterior brain involvement of Alzheimer's-type dementia evinces abnormalities in behavior of a more widespread pattern with frequent occurrences of delusions and hallucinations. Patterns of behavior in patients with frontotemporal dementia indicate greater disturbance but less depression than those observed with pure Alzheimer's dementia (Levy et al. 1997).

This is where advanced technology is essential because of the difficulty in clinically differentiating this dementia from Alzheimer's. A magnetic resonance imaging (MRI) scanner can readily distinguish between these two dementias by measuring the intensity of the white matter in the brain (Kitagaki et al. 1997).

Frontotemporal dementia is not reversible.

Pick's Disease

Pick's disease is a rare neurological disorder marked by a demyelenating process of the nerve sheaths (stripping of their coverings). It affects the front part of the brain and can sometimes be familial. Clinically, it manifests as personality deterioration and loss of memory, with its degenerative process affecting the hippocampus, the area also mainly involved in Alzheimer's.

Pick's disease is not reversible (Dickson 1998).

CHAPTER 5

Pathogenesis

CHANGES IN THE BRAIN

Major precipitating changes of Alzheimer's dementia are due to pathological (abnormal) alterations that cause amyloid, a protein normally found in brain tissue, to become toxic. It then begins to clump into formations known as beta-amyloid plaques. These plaques then act on nerve fibers in the brain, causing them to undergo secondary changes and evolve into injured, twisted, malformed tissue, known as neurofibrillary tangles and threads. Also referred to as "tombstones" and "ghosts," they signal nerve cell death (Grasby 1997).

A receptor named RAGE has been discovered on the surface of nerve cells by a research team headed by Dr. David Stern at Columbia University in New York and has been corroborated in other research centers. These neuronal receptors react with the toxic amyloid protein and trigger a reaction that causes nerve cell death. RAGE exists in very high amounts in the brain tissue of Alzheimer's patients (Yan et al. 1996).

A contrasting view suggests instead that the plaques are the result, rather than the cause, of Alzheimer's disease. This theory emerged when it was discovered that large amounts of abnormal plaque are found in significant numbers of people who do not have Alzheimer's. When brain cells die, secondary to a depletion of energy supplies such as a lack of oxygen, glucose, or metabolic disorders, there are fragments of mitochondria and compounds called "lysosomes" that comprise part of the plaque formations. Lysosomes are normally found within the brain's cellular structures and play a role similar to phagocytes (white blood cells responsible for attacking infection and foreign bodies) when a cell seriously breaks down. They release enzymes whose role is to dissolve the injured cells. This would explain why the pathogenesis of plaque formations are a result, rather than a cause, of cellular death (Blaylock 1996).

ALTERED NEUROTRANSMITTER SYSTEMS

There are greater than fifty neurotransmitter systems in the brain. These are pathways that control how impulses (messages) travel back and forth within the brain and between the brain and the rest of the body. Chemically, the neurotransmitters are amino acids or combinations of amino acids called peptides that, when combined in long chains, comprise the basic structure of protein. Each neurotransmitter serves a different function. Some are inhibitory (calming). Others are excitatory. Because the central nervous system is chemically under the control of amino acids, a significant deficiency of any one of these amino acids will adversely reflect the actions of its respective neurotransmitter.

Of the many neurotransmitters, there are three principal pathways that affect Alzheimer's patients: the cholinergic, the glutamine, and the tyrosine systems. A fourth neurotransmitter system, serotonin, has already been introduced and described in the explanation of depression.

The Acetylcholine Pathway

One pathway known as the choline, or cholinergic system, functions by a chemical neurotransmitter known as acetylcholine. Its primary purpose is to transmit nerve impulses across the nerve synapse (the connection between two nerves). A deficiency in acetylcholine results in a decrease or disruption of nerve transmission. When this involves the hippocampus, a particular segment of the brain, loss of memory and learning occurs due to the toxic brain protein plaquing that destroys this normal nerve pathway by inflicting injury and death upon the nerve cells.

Nontoxic amyloid protein can also destroy the cholinergic system by other mechanisms (Pedersen et al. 1996).

The percentage of loss of these neurotransmitters correlates directly to the severity of the dementia (Bierer et al. 1995). Cholinergic loss in the forebrain causes loss of attention. Drugs such as tacrine and nicotine that stimulate, or excite, the cholinergic system can significantly improve attention spans (Lawrence and Sahakian 1995).

The Glutamine Pathway

Another major neurotransmitter pathway involves the chemical glutamine. The salt of an amino acid known as glutamic acid, it interacts with learning and memory. Present in most areas of the brain, it is found in highest concentration in the hippocampus—the area of greatest involvement with Alzheimer's. Unlike acetylcholine, the body never lacks glutamine because it manufactures all that it needs and can even convert it from other amino acids such as aspartic acid, ornithine, arginine, and proline. Glutamic acid never needs supplementation. In fact, glutamic acid levels may actually increase for unknown reasons in some Alzheimer's patients, and this can cause seizures (Braverman et al. 1997a).

This glutamine nerve transmitter can be stimulated into an excitotoxin whereby the brain cell becomes hyperactive or "excited." This disrupts its metabolism as well as the transfer of its energy by the mitochondria, thus resulting in cell death. Degeneration of nerve cells significantly increases when toxic amyloid protein combines with glutamine (Gray and Patel 1995).

The Tyrosine Pathway

The essential amino acid tyrosine is a cardinal ingredient in several other neurotransmitter pathways in the brain. It is the precursor of the neurotransmitters *dopamine, norepinephrine,* and *epinephrine* (adrenaline). Deficiencies of these three neurotransmitters are typically found in Alzheimer's patients, and supplementation with tyrosine can prevent further damage to these neurotransmitter systems.

Tyrosine has other major roles besides the manufacture of neurotransmitters:

- It is found inside a protein located within brain cells and is necessary for the structure of these brain cells.
- It guards against fatigue.
- It plays a significant role in the treatment of depression by maintaining high levels of dopamine. This is particularly beneficial to that subgroup of patients suffering from "dopamine dependent depression"

Essential for the integrity of neurotransmitters and brain cell structure and effective against fatigue and depression, tyrosine is believed to be the most important stress-relieving nutrient recognized in medicine. Foods high in tyrosine are wild game, pork, cottage cheese, and ricotta cheese. (Braverman et al. 1997b).

Tyrosine is a crucial element in the prevention of Alzheimer's. Supplements are available in health food and grocery stores and recommended at 1 to 2 g daily.

Patients taking MAOI class of drugs or diagnosed with schizophrenia should avoid tyrosine supplementation.

FREE RADICAL DAMAGE

It is now universally accepted that free radical damage is a significant cause of Alzheimer's disease, as well as a major contributor in heart disease, stroke, aging, and depressed immune systems. Free radicals are, in part, responsible for toxic plaque formation and excitotoxicity of neurons (nerve cells), thus creating a wide range of cellular metabolic disorders. When mitochondrial derangement occurs due to the disruption of electron transport (energy), the mitochondria (control mechanisms for each cell) cannot function and survive. Free radicals, combined with oxidative stress, are responsible for brain cell degeneration.

Abnormal energy metabolism causes amyloidosis (inflammation of the amyloid protein) that effects pathologic changes in cellular structure resulting in damage to the neuron and disruption of its energy output. Disrupted energy production causes abnormal calcium metabolism in brain cells, interruption of cholinergic neurotransmission, and loss of nerve cells and synapses (Blass 1996).

Antioxidants are known to slow down the development of Alzheimer's dementia by fighting these free radicals. Inhibition or removal of these free radicals can reverse neurotoxicity, a major process that damages nerve cells. This fact strengthens the theory that free radicals play a decisive role in the pathogenesis (abnormal tissue changes) of Alzheimer's (Frolich and Riederer 1995; Thome et al. 1997). This readily explains why supplementation with vitamin E, a potent antioxidant and anti-inflammatory agent, is so highly effective in slowing the progression as well as preventing Alzheimer's when started early in the disease process.

Studies at Case Western Reserve University indicate that the combination of free radical scavengers, antioxidants, and elimination of iron are effective against Alzheimer's (Smith and Perry 1995).

OXIDATIVE STRESS

Oxidative stress, like free radical damage, is an abnormal metabolic reaction responsible for plaque deposition and neurofibrillary tangles. It plays a major role in cellular brain death. In fact, disturbance of the free radical mechanism can lead to oxidative stress and Alzheimer's dementia (Thome et al. 1997).

ELECTRON TRANSPORT DISORDERS

Disorder of the electron transport system is rapidly gaining increased acceptance as a direct pathogenic element of Alzheimer's. When fat and sugar are metabolized (oxidized), they produce energy that fuels the electron transport system and the mitochondria. The mechanics of mitochondrial damage and disruption of electron transfer (energy) are compared to the mechanics of a computer. If the electric current isn't transported properly, the computer can lose stored memory or functions from its brain, or, if extensive enough, the entire system can shut down.

Because the mitochondria govern the manufacture of ATP, a chemical that is the primary energy source for the conduction of nerve impulses, and because damage to the mitochondria by free oxygen radicals disrupts the electron transfer system, cells die when mitochondria are unable to function. This is believed to be a significant predisposing factor in the pathogenesis leading to Alzheimer's.

The discovery by Dr. John Walker that disruption in the electron transport system contributes to aging (for which he was awarded the Nobel Prize) is identical to the same changes responsible for the development of Alzheimer's (Walker and Kmietowicz 1997). Electron transport disruption results in the formation of free radicals, excitotoxicity reactants, and damage from oxidative stress (Klivenyi and Vescei 1997; Beal 1996).

COENZYME Q10 TO THE RESCUE

Disruption of the electron pathway (energy production) must be prevented to avoid damage to the mitochondria and neuronal death. Coenzyme Q10, a chemical normally found in small amounts in the body, is rapidly emerging as a very effective preventive measure against this component of Alzheimer's disease. Coenzyme Q10 acts upon the mitochondria of every cell of the body, enhances the electron transport system, and corrects dysfunctions in the brain and every other organ system in the body.

The role of coenzyme Q10 in the treatment of Alzheimer's is certain. To summarize, for basic survival brain cells require energy; this energy is produced by ATP. The metabolism of ATP and transport of this energy are governed by the mitochondria. When a cell is injured or damaged by toxic amyloid plaquing, excitotoxicity, oxidative stress, or free radical damage, these pathological processes impinge upon the mitochondria, inflammation results, and a powerful antidote is immediately required. Coenzyme Q10 not only meets this challenge, but, when used as a supplement, it can continually bathe the cells of the brain to help prevent the mitochondria from becoming damaged and guard the brain against the development of Alzheimer's.

CHAPTER 6

Causes

Numerous and varied entities are constantly being proposed as potential causes of Alzheimer's disease. Many of them have been irrefutably accepted. Others are currently under investigation but not yet thoroughly evaluated. Some will be proven incorrect, while others, totally unknown today, will gain prominence as research continues. The most up-to-date research in all categories of precursors and causes is presented here.

BACTERIAL INFECTION

To date, evaluation of infectious causes of Alzheimer's has focused on viral diseases such as herpes simplex (fever blisters), herpes zoster (shingles), and Creutzfeldt-Jakob (mad cow disease). Recent discoveries reveal bacterial infection as a probable cause of Alzheimer's.

Chlamydia pneumoniae, a common bacterial infection of the nose, sinuses, and lungs, has been found and isolated from the brains of Alzheimer's patients. A chronic infection such as this would account for the chronic inflammatory changes found in Alzheimer's patients. Research teams from three universities, including the Alzheimer's Disease Ressearch Center at Johns Hopkins University in Baltimore, recovered this bacteria from seventeen of nineteen patients who were evaluated for bacterial infection at the time of autopsy.

LOW BLOOD SUGAR (HYPOGLYCEMIA)

Low blood sugar, known as hypoglycemia, can be a precursor of Alzheimer's. Statistically, individuals with low blood sugar have nearly twice as much chance of developing Alzheimer's dementia as the normal population.

Conversely, individuals with high blood sugar (diabetes) have a lesser incidence of developing Alzheimer's. The risk of Alzheimer's in diabetics is approximately one-half that of the normal population.

Brain Damage

Temporary lack of glucose to the brain (hypoglycemia) is known to cause abnormal metabolism, mitochondrial damage, disruption of energy flow, and cell death. These pathological disruptions can occur sporadically at any time during life, beginning as early as the fetal stage. Although genetics is suspected as being a prominent factor in the development of hypoglycemia, refined sugar aggravates the condition because the initial elevation in blood sugar after eating simple sugars (sweets) is followed by an equal and opposite rebound drop in blood sugar two hours later, creating a hypoglycemic state in both blood and brain. Even a crash diet has the potential of causing some small degree of cellular brain death due to a lack of sugar and corresponding deficiency energy production. Although there are billions of neurons in the brain, recurrent, irreversible, and asymptomatic episodes of cellular death over many years' duration may eventually exact its toll—a slow progression of Alzheimer's.

Abnormal Glucose Metabolism

Abnormal glucose metabolism lowers a person's blood sugar levels, and its decreased availability in the brain causes memory impairment. This fact is now accepted as one of the origins of Alzheimer's. Therefore, it might be logical that when blood sugar levels are raised, increasing its availability in the brain, an Alzheimer's patient's memory should improve.

Insulin Levels

The increase in blood sugar causes a secondary elevation in blood insulin levels. Speculation continues regarding as to whether improved memory status in Alzheimer's patients is due to increased availability of sugar to the brain, or is instead due to increased levels of insulin acting on brain tissue totally independent of elevated sugar levels. The presence of insulin receptors in the hippocampus explains the suspected mechanism for this improved memory. A striking increase in memory is noted when blood sugar is kept at a fasting (but not hypoglycemic) state and insulin levels are elevated (Craft and Newcomer 1996).

Another study to determine if insulin levels can actually affect memory found that Alzheimer's patients had lower levels of insulin in the cerebrospinal fluid of the brain and higher levels in the blood compared to healthy adults. As the disease progresses, these differences become more extreme (Craft et al. 1998). Clinically, lower levels of insulin in the brain appear to decrease memory, whereas higher levels increase memory.

Treatment of Hypoglycemia

Short- and Long-Chain Starches

Dietary control is the standard treatment for hypoglycemia (low blood sugar). It involves:

- avoidance of short-chain carbohydrates or simple starches (simple sugars)
- use of long-chain carbohydrates (complex sugars) by complex carbohydrates
- smaller but more frequent meals
- use of dietary soluble fiber

Simple sugars (sweets) are defined as processed sugars and their manmade products, such as cane sugar, maple syrup, jellies, syrups, candies, pastries, pies, ice cream, carbonated drinks, and all those other foodstuffs that rot away our teeth. On the other hand, complex carbohydrates are the long-chain starches (the good sugars) such as whole grain cereals, unrefined breads, and brown rice. The intermediate starches such as legumes (peas, beans) and the other starchy vegetables (corn, yams, potatoes, etc.) are okay because they are broken down and absorbed more slowly and evenly than simple sugars, thus avoiding the rapid rise and corresponding rapid, decline in blood sugar.

Sir Isaac Newton's Law of Thermodynamics states that "for every action there is an equal and opposite reaction." This law holds true for most things in life, particularly blood sugar, since the higher blood sugar elevates following a meal, the lower it will drop, creating a hypoglycemic state in both blood and brain between one and two hours after eating. The low blood sugar reaction, therefore, can be avoided by eating both intermediate and long-chain starches because they are broken down and metabolized much more slowly in the body, avoiding the wide pendulumlike swings in blood sugar levels.

Frequent Meals

Dividing each day's three planned meals into four to six meals, being careful to avoid increasing the total daily calorie count, and complying with the regimen of eating long-chain carbohydrates instead of simple sugars and sweets, will avoid those blood sugar swings that lead to hypoglycemia.

Dietary Fiber

There are two kinds of fiber: one is water soluble, the other is not.

The water-soluble fibers like psyllium seed (Metamucil), pectin (apples, oranges, grapefruit), oat bran, and guar gum effectively delay the absorption and transport of sugar into the bloodstream, thereby reducing the amount of insulin required (Wakabayashi 1992). This prevents the rapid rise and corresponding drop in blood sugar after eating (hypoglycemia). The water-soluble fibers can decrease the chances of Alzheimer's by aiding in bowel regulation, lowering serum cholesterol and reducing atherosclerosis, thereby further reducing the chances of developing Alzheimer's and vascular dementias.

The nonsoluble fibers such as wheat fiber, rice bran, some vegetables and fruits, and other gums do not delay the absorption of sugars from the gut nor do they afford the same degree of protection against cholesterol. They do contain laxative properties, however.

Sugar-beet fiber is certainly important because it elevates HDL-cholesterol concentration significantly by 12 percent, lowers fasting total cholesterol concentrations by 8.5 percent, and lowers fasting LDL-cholesterol concentrations by 9.6 percent (Frape and Jones 1995).

The Dual Role of Chromium

Chromium supplementation at a recommended dosage of 100 to 200 mcg twice daily is helpful in regulating insulin resistance and improving low blood sugar. Side effects are virtually nonexistent, even at levels of 600 and 800 mg. Many diabetic patients can also benefit from chromium supplementation because it may allow them to decrease or eliminate oral insulin doses.

Chromium seems to decrease body fat and increase muscle mass. It promotes significant activity on the regression of atherosclerotic plaques in experimental mice (Abraham et al. 1980) and may play a role in longevity as shown by its ability to increase by one-third the life span of experimental rats.

Adult Onset Diabetes

Hypoglycemia can persist throughout a person's lifetime. In one subset of hypoglycemic patients, blood sugars slowly escalated with aging, and many developed adult onset diabetes. We would expect the progressive risk of developing Alzheimer's to lessen in this subset as their blood sugar levels rise.

Hypoglycemia Symptoms

The varied symptoms of hypoglycemia include shakiness, cyclic tiredness, daytime hypersomnolence (sleepiness), hunger, irritability, sweats, migraines, insomnia (inability to sleep at night), dizziness, and mental confusion. Such symptoms are usually relieved by eating a small amount of something sweet.

Hypoglycemia does not always follow expected patterns. Be on the alert for unexpected and marked deviations in symptoms. If blood sugar drops too low, the milder symptom of hypersomnolence can progress into seizures and unconsciousness. Blood sugar levels normally range from 70 to 110 mg percent. Below 70 mg percent is considered low. The lower the sugar level, the greater the chances and severity of symptoms. Mild symptoms may generally be seen in the low 60s or high 50s. It is not unknown for patients suffering from grand mal seizures and a misdiagnosis of epilepsy to actually be having seizures primarily the result of severely depressed blood sugar in the low 40s or high 30s. Cellular brain damage is significantly increased at these critically low levels due to glucose deprivation. On the other hand, I have seen patients with levels in the 40s who were completely devoid of symptoms. This is the realm in which hypoglycemia can perform the greatest amount of damage because an atypical presentation of recurrent and chronic episodes of totally undetected hypoglycemia will remain untreated over many years and a slow but unrelenting toll in the death of neurons (brain cells).

Whether from hypoglycemic episodes, TIAs, or other insults to the brain and the mitochondria in particular, dysfunction of electron transfer, and decreased energy production by the mitochondria result in rapid cell death (Blaylock 1996) and is a significant cause of Alzheimer's.

STRESS

Prolonged and chronic psychological stress (home, work, financial, etc.) can induce Alzheimer's (Hull et al. 1996b) independent of any inflammatory origin. This theory is based on the following data: a chemical called interleukin-6, believed to be induced by an inflammatory mechanism within the brain is found in Alzheimer's brains, mostly in the toxic plaques before neurofibrillary changes take place. However, it is not found in the brains of nondemented control groups. Its synthesis is prevented and/or suppressed by treating brain cells with anti-inflammatory agents. Psychological stress seems to trigger production of interleukin-6 (Bauer and Hull 1995).

Stress can lower the immune system and contribute to heart attacks. We know that stress increases the production of adrenaline and steroids, causes decreased production of white blood cells that attack infection, and causes the thymus gland to shrink. The thymus is therefore unable to fully conduct its proper role to produce sufficient numbers of T cells that also attack infection. This may explain why caregivers have higher rates of infections than do noncaregivers.

Further research and evaluation about how stress contributes to the development of Alzheimer's are needed.

HEAD INJURY

Head Trauma

Head trauma, especially with injuries involving a loss of consciousness, definitely contributes to the development of Alzheimer's. Several studies have shown that a history of head injuries is far more prevalent in Alzheimer's patients than in their healthy elderly counterparts.

1995). Blocking this H_2 type of histamine prevents brain cell injury and death. Thus it delays the onset and possibly prevents development of Alzheimer's.

ANTIHISTAMINES

Some antihistamines can either contribute to or exacerbate Alzheimer's. Normally prescribed to counteract and control allergic reactions, they are designed to prevent release of the H_1 type of histamine that creates the allergic reaction (not to be confused with H_2, above). Several antihistamines exhibit other properties, however. Some calm the nerves and thus function as anxiolytics (antianxiety) agents or tranquilizers. One agent that has been in wide use for many years as an anxiolytic is the antihistamine chlorpromazine (Thorazine), which appears to play a role in Alzheimer's disease.

Aside from the once-scorned but significanly effective herbal medicines, barbituates were the only known tranquilizers in this country in the 1950s. The development of the first major tranquilizer, Equanil (meprobamate) by Wyeth Pharmaceuticals in Philadelphia, Pennsylvania, was an astounding success. Indeed, it revolutionized the treatment of nerves and anxiety and sparked a stampede for anxiolytics by other pharmaceutical companies. In the rush to market new products, some of the first anxiolytics were actually basic antihistaminic formulas such as Vistaril (Atarax), Phenergan (promethazine), and Thorazine (chlorpromazine).

Present research reveals that prolonged use of Thorazine can contribute to the development of Alzheimer's because it acts against the cholinergic neurotransmitting system. What adverse effects other antihistamines might have in contributing to Alzheimer's can only be speculated upon at this time (Oken 1995).

MEDICATIONS

Choline is the building block of the neurotransmitter acetylcholine, and cholinergic nerve transmitters are located in the cerebral hemisphere of the brain. Any substance or medicine that supports the cholinergic role in the brain will help keep this system healthy and guard against Alzheimer's. Conversely, any substance or medicine that fights against the cholinergic pathways (acetylcholine) in the brain, even though potentially beneficial to other body organ systems, has the potential to cause harm to brain cells (Oken 1995). Prolonged or indiscriminate use of anti- cholinergic medication such as Thorazine, Bentyl, or Donnatal has the potential to cause harm to the brain's neurotransmitting system.

ELECTROMAGNETIC FIELDS

Electromagnetism in the environment, sometimes accused as a contributing factor in various cancers, is now also suspected as a possible cause of Alzheimer's. Independent controlled studies at the University of Southern California and in Helsinki, Finland, have revealed that the mechanism by which electromagnetic exposure works is the disruption of the immune system cells in the brain, thereby setting the stage for the breakdown and death of nerve cells (Sobel et al. 1995). Common sources of low-grade exposures in the home and workplace are hair dryers, electric blankets, cellular phones, electric shavers, and microwave ovens.

SOLVENT EXPOSURE

Research at the University of Washington implicates present and prior exposure to several groups of organic solvents including benzene, toluene, and ketones as possible causes of Alzheimer's (Kukull et al. 1995). Toluene, in particular, is used in the construction industry, and it can trigger some rather severe symptoms such as vertigo (dizziness), nausea, vomiting, asthma, muscle weakness, marked fatigue, and mental confusion if the newly constructed area is insufficiently ventilated. Caution must be exercised to avoid skin contact, swallowing, or inhaling these solvents.

CHRONIC INFLAMMATION AND ANTI-INFLAMMATORY MEDICINES

Anti-inflammatory medications such as ibuprofen are able to delay the onset of Alzheimer's symptoms for prolonged periods of time. This indicates that an apparent underlying chronic inflammatory process may indeed be a cause of dementia. A low-grade inflammatory state is a trigger mechanism for toxifying amyloid protein and for hyperexciting the neurotransmitter glutamine.

Inflammation

Compelling evidence reveals inflammation is a definite cause rather than a result of Alzheimer's (Rogers 1995). A fourteen-year study of over 2,000 elderly people indicated that taking anti-inflammatories reduces the risk of developing Alzheimer's by as much as 60 percent. The longer the period of time anti-inflammatories are taken, the lower the incidence of developing Alzheimer's. Although ibuprofen was the agent used in the study, other anti-inflammatory agents are also effective. Aspirin and Tylenol, however, do not protect against Alzheimer's disease (Stewart et al. 1996). Anti-inflammatory medications now play a major role in the fight against Alzheimer's and should be an integral part of any treatment plan.

Chronic inflammation in the brain is a well-documented cause of autotoxic (self-destructive) damage to brain cells. Inflammatory states in other areas of the body are also known to cause abnormal changes in the brain. Thus, inflammation both within the brain and in distant sites can be responsible for cellular death by toxic plaque deposition and excitotoxic changes.

Brain Markers

Interleukin-6, a chemical associated with inflammation, is found in the brains of Alzheimer's subjects but is absent in elderly controls who are not demented. It is also implicated in prolonged and chronic stress (Bauer and Hull 1995). The appearance of interleukin-6 and the resultant inflammatory response actually precede the development of brain plaquing and nerve degeneration. Psychological stress, as previously described, is also observed to generate interleukin-6 (Hull et al. 1996b).

Self-Destruction

Certain types of brain cells called microglia rise to kill off infection but become their own worst enemy by inducing further nerve cell damage as they proliferate. When the toxic beta-amyloid protein is deposited in clumps, it creates an "acute phase response" in this degenerating process. During this acute phase, defensive media-tors are produced to enhance the anti-inflammatory and immune systems to fight off inflammation and infection. It is at this point that the brain's microglia activate. These brain cells act the way white blood cells do when they attack infection: they phagocytize (eat up) foreign bodies like bacteria and viruses. The action of these microglia, however, can be counterproductive because they gener-ate oxygen radicals and proteolytic enzymes that cause greater damage to brain cells (Kalaria 1996).

The Power of Anti-inflammatories

Numerous studies indicate that taking anti-inflammatories can decrease risk of developing Alzheimer's. In a preliminary clinical trial, Indocin (indomethacin) has been shown to actually arrest the progress (McGeer and McGeer 1995). This and many other kinds of anti-inflammatories work to reduce and prevent the death of inflamed neurons caused by excitotoxicity, toxic beta-amyloid, proliferation of microglia, and interleukin-6.

CHRONIC VIRAL INFECTION

Creutzfeldt-Jakob disease (mad cow disease) is a low-grade, chronic viral infection that targets the brain and causes changes similar to the damage found in Alzheimer's disease. The clinical symptoms of mad cow disease present as a chronic fatigue–like syndrome followed by wasting and dementia, thereby mimicking

Alzheimer's symptoms. Because of these similarities, a low-grade, chronic viral infection is now suspected as a possible cause of Alzheimer's. The amount of apolipoprotein E is increased in the brains of Alzheimer's and Creutzfeldt-Jakob patients and not in normal brain specimens (Aizawa et al. 1997).

Both Alzheimer's and mad cow disease exhibit the pathological brain changes of amyloidosis, an inflammation of the amyloid protein that produces the same toxic plaques normally found in pure Alzheimer's (Barcikowska et al. 1995). The disease is transmitted when an animal eats fodder made from "should-have-been-discarded" ground-up body parts of diseased slaughtered cows. Mad cow disease is then transferable to humans who consume the infected beef. Alzheimer's is not transferable, however.

HERPES SIMPLEX VIRUS INFECTION

Skin, Mouth, or Brain?

Herpes simplex virus type 1 (HSV 1) is responsible for the common fever blister. Usually limited to the mucous membranes of the mouth and lips, it can involve any skin surface. This lesion has been tagged "fever blister" because it frequently accompanies fever or any infection. This virus is an opportunist and will attack whenever the hosts resistance is down. Lowered resistance does not have to be an infection since the virus routinely gains a foothold with physical stress and emotional stress, and even recurs monthly with menstrual cycles. Brain involvement is quite infrequent and it may occur only once, but it can be many times in subsequent years.

APOE 4 and Herpes: The Danger Zone

Herpes infection by itself, no matter how repetitive it is, is not a cause of Alzheimer's. The combination of this virus infecting the brain plus the host's possession of the apolipoprotein E4 gene (APOE 4) is a strong risk factor for developing Alzheimer's, however. Those patients already diagnosed with Alzheimer's and APOE 4 who harbor a latent form of HSV 1 involving the brain do face greater neuronal damage with reactivation of the virus (Itzhaki et al. 1997). Many patients exhibiting mild symptoms such as a low-grade fever, chills, generalized muscle aching, and headache that lasts for several days may not seek medical attention and are often totally unaware that the symptoms may be due to a mild herpes viral meningitis.

Of this very small but significant segment of the population, people with APOE 4 are at greater risk for Alzheimer's (Lin, Shang, and Itzhaki 1996).

SHINGLES

A study of a small group of five patients who suffered over many years from a progressive dementia clinically identical to Alzheimer's showed surprising findings at autopsy. Four of five cases evaluated possessed no pathological brain findings of Alzheimer's. Instead, their findings were compatible with previous viral encephalitis of herpetic origin. Prior histories revealed three cases of herpes zoster (shingles) of the skin and one case of viral meningoencephalitis (brain infection).

Herpes zoster is a first cousin to the herpes simplex virus. It produces a nasty, painful, red-violet, blistering, and scabbing rash on the skin. But its primary pathology is against nerves, and it follows the pathway of the nerves it attacks. The skin lesions indicative of herpes zoster, commonly known as shingles, are far more painful than herpes simplex, and the patient can be left with pain for years after the blisters are gone.

In each of these cases studied, memory loss started at the same time as the reported infection. The fifth case presented an Alzheimer's-related dementia known as sclerosis. The study indicated that repeated reactivation of the herpes zoster virus may link it to the Alzheimer's type of dementia (Ball, Kaye, and Steiner 1997). Since no actual Alzheimer's lesions were identified, these new findings will now relegate shingles dementia to the classification of "Alzheimer's-related dementias."

THIAMINE DEFICIENCY

Thiamine (vitamin B_1) is essential to the function and survival of brain cells because of its role in several chemical reactions and enzyme functions. A deficiency can result in Alzheimer's dementia. Autopsy reveals disruption of these thiamine-dependent chemical reactions (Heroux et al. 1996).

Thiamine protects the mitochondria against the oxidative stress responsible for neuronal death, and its deficiency results in decline and loss of cognition. Treatment of Alzheimer's patients with thiamine derivatives results in improved emotions and intellectual function (Mimori, Katsuoka, and Nakamura 1996).

AMINO ACID DEFICIENCIES

Amino acids, the basic structures of all neurotransmitters and the building blocks of all proteins, are deficient in Alzheimer's patients although they remain normal in age-matched controls. The amino acids tryptophan and methionine are significantly decreased in the early stages of Alzheimer's while their levels remain normal in the control groups. It is suspected that these lowered levels are responsible for changes in behavior that are seen in the later stages of Alzheimer's (Fekkes et al. 1998).

HOMOCYSTEINE ELEVATION

The amino acid homocysteine is one of several recognized causes of atherosclerosis (hardening of the arteries) and heart attacks when present at excessive levels. It is also an acknowledged cause of a neurological abnormality in newborn babies that results in an embryonic neural tube deficit responsible for a protrusion of the spinal cord known as spina bifida.

The latest discovery of elevated homocysteine levels in Alzheimer's patients compared to normal controls implicates it as a cause of Alzheimer's disease. Furthermore, the elevated homocysteine level is accompanied by a deficiency in folic acid (a B-complex vitamin), and supplementing the diet with folic acid reverses an elevated homocysteine level toward normal. In addition, vitamin B_{12} deficiency is now suspected to contribute to high homocysteine levels (McCaddon et al. 1998).

VITAMIN E DEFICIENCY

It is increasingly evident that Alzheimer's patients lack vitamin E, as seen in lowered levels with laboratory testing and by significant response to clinical treatment. Concentrations of vitamin E, vitamin A, and beta-carotene are all significantly reduced in Alzheimer's patients (Zaman et al. 1992; Toghi et al. 1994). A study at the Salk Institute reveals that vitamin E protects brain cells from glutamate toxicity by means of its antioxidant and free radical scavenging properties (Behl et al. 1992).

Numerous studies demonstrate that the progression of dementia can be delayed—even into late stages— with supplemental vitamin E intake. Intervention early enough in the course of the disease both delays the onset of Alzheimer's and can actually help prevent it.

HORMONAL DEFICIENCIES

Hormone deficiencies may be implicated as components of the pathological changes that lead to the development of Alzheimer's disease. As we age, hormones such as DHEA, melatonin, nerve growth factor, and estrogen are known to diminish significantly. The damaging effects of insufficiency and the potential benefits of replacing these hormones are areas of ongoing intensive scientific research. Estrogen replacement therapy has already proven to be markedly effective against Alzheimer's. Nerve growth factor is currently under investigation and holds significant promise in terms of growth, protection, and even regeneration of nerve cells. Melatonin also possesses several important properties that are important to Alzheimer's patients, while the efficacy of DHEA is still being evaluated.

Estrogen

Estrogen replacement provides a 55 percent reduction in the risk of developing Alzheimer's disease, according to the results of the "Baltimore Longitudinal Study" at the Alzheimer's Disease Research Center and the National Institute of Aging and Johns Hopkins University (Kawas et al. 1997). Obviously, the crucial role it plays relates to females, and it provides many remarkable benefits.

Estrogen has also proven effective in males by lowering homocysteine and fibrinogen, causing factors in heart attacks, and in elevating HDL, the "good cholesterol," thus providing protection for the heart in males just as it does in women (Giri et al. 1998). To date no beneficial effects have been found that suggest protection against Alzheimer's in men, and I am unaware of any ongoing studies. However, eating a cup of soy per day or drinking soymilk, thereby supplying the natural phytoestrogen equivalent of a Premarin tablet, theoretically provides the same protection against Alzheimer's in men as it does in women.

Nerve Growth Factor

Research on mice over the past decade has enabled us to genetically transform these rodents by implanting an abnormal gene that promotes a linkage to a type of Alzheimer's. Known as transgenic mice, they evince learning and memory problems similar to humans, but their genetically linked learning and memory loss is completely reversed and restored by the administration of nerve growth factor (NGF) which completely reverses cell shrinkage (Phillips et al. 1997). Thus, NGF shows considerable promise for the prevention and treatment of Alzheimer's by restoration of function and reversal of Alzheimer's symptoms.

Melatonin

Melatonin is an amino acid that performs as a hormone. It functions as an antioxidant, a hydroxyl radical scavenger, and a neurotransmitter, while regulating circadian rhythms. There is a significant lack of melatonin in Alzheimer's patients compared to their normal counterparts. It has a definite place in the treatment of Alzheimer's disease, especially as it relates to sundowner's syndrome since melatonin can reset the mixed-up internal day-night clock known as circadian rhythm (Maurizi 1995).

DHEA and DHEA-S (Over-the-Counter)

DHEA (dehydroepiandrosterone), known as the "Mother Hormone," is the precursor of several other hormones including estrogen and testosterone. DHEA levels drop considerably during aging—as much as 48 percent lower in Alzheimer's patients, in fact, compared to their "normal" counterparts. Its efficacy as a supplement is unclear in Alzheimer's disease, even though it is strongly proving its importance in other areas.

As to the role it plays in Alzheimer's, a decrease in the concentration of its sulfate form, DHEA-S (dehydroepiandrosterone sulfate), is recognized. Since the level of DHEA is decreased in other dementias also, its possible significance in the treatment of Alzheimer's is unclear (Yanase 1996). DHEA supplementation provides greater protection in guarding against atherosclerosis (hardening of the arteries), heart attacks, and possibly prostate cancer than it might appear to in Alzheimer's, but its marked decline in Alzheimer's disease is accompanied by a corresponding increase in the deposition of beta-amyloid, thus suggesting a strong correlation between the deficiency of DHEA and the pathogenesis of Alzheimer's (Danenberg et al. 1995). In another study, DHEA was not found to combat Alzheimer's. However, its sulfated derivative, DHEA-S, was found to be neuroprotective, specifically protecting the nerve cells in the hippocampus from glutamate toxic excitation (Mao and Barger 1998).

HEAVY METALS

Aluminum

Excess aluminum has been implicated as a major cause of Alzheimer's disease because numerous autopsy studies have shown aluminum deposits in the affected areas of brains of Alzheimer's patients. It has also been implicated in memory loss, mood swings, and seizures.

It is nearly impossible to avoid constant exposure. Aluminum compounds can be absorbed by foods and then ingested by our body. We cook in aluminum utensils, package foods in aluminum containers, store leftovers in aluminum foil, and use aluminum in underarm deodorants. Most antacids contain aluminum. It is even found in some douches, shampoos, and antidiarrheal medication. It is present in infant immunization injections. Low levels of aluminum are found in drinking water. At high levels it might have a definite causal relationship to Alzheimer's (Forbes and McLachlan 1996).

According to an article released by the Alzheimer's Association titled "The Aluminum Association's Statement on Aluminum and Health," a fifteen-year study by the Aluminum Association has exonerated aluminum as a causative factor in the development of Alzheimer's. This stance, moreover, has been supported by the National Institutes of Health, the U.S. Food and Drug Administration, the World Health Organization, the U.S. Environmental Protection Agency, and the Alzheimer's Association. Their logic is that there is not enough evidence to include aluminum as a causative factor.

Controversy exists nevertheless. A study at Wakayama Medical College in Japan revealed a significant increase in the amount of aluminum as well as iron in Alzheimer's patients compared to controls, suggesting a role in pathogenesis (Yoshida and Yoshimasu 1996). A study at Aston University in Birmingham, England, indicates that aluminum in vaccines created a chemical reaction that could cause amyloid plaquing and nerve death (Armstrong, Winsper, and Blair 1995). After giving countless immunization shots containing aluminum to infants over years, I question if the medical profession, albeit well intentioned, might not have actually caused some minor, unknown damage.

A Department of Health Study at the University of Waterloo, Ontario, Canada, revealed a possible link between high levels of aluminum in drinking water and incidence of Alzheimer's (Forbes and McLachlan 1996). Conversely, a study in Oslo, Norway, revealed no statistical differences at autopsy in the amounts of bulk aluminum between Alzheimer's patients and normal controls (Bjertness et al. 1996).

Aluminum is also implicated in a damaging chemical reaction against blood platelets, those tiny, flat, coinlike structures in the bloodstream that are involved in normal clotting. Aluminum causes lipid peroxidation of their membranes (cell wall coverings), the abnormal metabolism of the fat comprising part of the membrane walls of every cell of the body (Daniels et al. 1998). Controversy obviously continues. The aluminum door remains ajar.

Mercury

There is also controversy about the role of mercury. Mercury in dental fillings is implicated as a cause of Alzheimer's. Fish from contaminated waters can contain high levels of heavy metals that may indeed be a causative factor. One recent study at the University of Nebraska, however, showed no significant increase of brain mercury in Alzheimer's patients over controls. The study was unable to substantiate claims that mercury contributes to the pathogenesis of Alzheimer's (Fung et al. 1997).

Zinc

Among the heavy metals, zinc is now a primary suspect as a potential source of Alzheimer's.

A test performed by Dr. Y. Tanzi at Harvard University involved the addition of zinc to amyloid protein (the one found normally in the brain) in a test tube. The protein clumped in a manner similar to that seen in autopsy findings of Alzheimer's brains.

A study at the University of Kentucky revealed a significant increase in both iron and zinc and a significant decrease in copper in the hippocampus. These changes result in severe tissue alteration at autopsy in Alzheimer's patients (Deibel, Ehrmann, and Markesberry 1996).

Zinc has a high affinity for binding to amyloid protein and can act as a toxin by aggregating the beta-amyloid protein and leading to plaque formation (Esler et al. 1996). There are numerous studies confirming this strong affinity for zinc to bond to amyloid and is neurotoxic at high concentrations (Cuajungco and Lees 1997), which essentially means that it is poisonous to brain cells and can cause injury.

Excessive supplementation of zinc, well above normal blood levels, is also implicated in heart disease. Numerous studies over several years now indicate that too much zinc causes the level of HDL (the good cholesterol) to sharply decrease, and LDL (the bad cholesterol), total cholesterol levels, and triglycerides to rise, thus promoting incidence of atherosclerosis (hardening of the arteries) (Hooper et al. and 1980; Hiller et al. 1995).

To summarize, as excess of zinc can:

- have a toxic involvement with beta-amyloid causing plaque formation in the brain, thereby accelerating Alzheimer's
- increase total cholesterol
- increase LDL (the bad cholesterol)
- decrease HDL (the good cholesterol)
- increase blood platelet aggregation and clot formation
- foster atherogenesis if levels are excessive

Conversely, zinc replacement in deficiency states engenders complementary activity in the skin and the male prostate gland, where it is found in the greatest amounts. Clinically, it is a standard and time-honored adjunctive treatment to control acute prostatitis and BPH (benign prostatic hypertrophy—"the old man's disease"), a hardening and swelling of the prostate gland that obstructs urine flow.

When there is a deficiency of zinc, a person's immune response is seriously depressed. T cells and B cells, the essential antibody response to infection and cancer, are reduced, and the body's natural killer cells are decreased (Ripa and Ripa 1994). A compromised immune system, in turn, can generate the injurious effects that cause Alzheimer's.

The beneficial properties of zinc (at normal levels) include:

- It is an antioxidant and protects against Alzheimer's.
- It prevents the oxidation of LDL, thus protecting against heart disease and stroke.
- It is a free radical scavenger; it blocks the pathological changes caused by free oxygen radicals (Bagchi, Bagchi, and Stohs 1997), and further protects against Alzheimer's.
- It is deficient in people with high blood pressure, and replacement restores blood pressure to normal (Ripa and Ripa 1994b).
- It blocks certain calcium actions that favor atherogenesis and Alzheimer's.
- A deficiency severely depresses the immune response (Ripa and Ripa 1995), and replacement restores immune function.
- Zinc levels decrease as we become older and require replacement.

Normal blood and tissue levels of zinc exert several beneficial roles, while both deficiencies and excesses are harmful. It can either help prevent or accelerate Alzheimer's. When taking supplemental zinc to treat certain disease states or replace deficiencies, caution must be exercised against excessive amounts or taking it for unnecessarily prolonged periods since blood and tissue levels that are too high can cause the harmful effects described above.

Iron

If untreated, too much iron in the blood causes hemochromatosis, an uncommon but potentially fatal disease, the opposite of anemia. Excess iron causes a marked overproduction of free radicals that are harmful to every organ system in the body. Known to cause severe and even fatal liver damage, evidence also indicates its involvement with Alzheimer's due to its free radical activity.

Numerous reports increasingly implicate iron with involvement in the pathogenesis (abnormal causative changes) of Alzheimer's. There is a cross-linking of proteins and amino acids in the brain, and these combine with heavy metals, such as iron, to produce oxygen radicals that cause cellular membrane damage (Smith, Sayre, and Perry 1996). Iron acts as a free radical, and it is involved in oxidative stress, both known factors in the pathogenesis of Alzheimer's.

An iron-binding protein is significantly increased in the blood of Alzheimer's patients compared to their normal counterparts so it can function as a marker for disease (Kennard et al. 1996). By testing for this protein, we are able to identify and follow the progress of Alzheimer's. Several studies, including M. A. Deibel's work at the University of Kentucky, indicated severe hippocampal tissue changes at autopsy accompanied by significant elevations of iron and zinc.

Tin

Tin levels are elevated in Alzheimer's patients. Experimental animals that are given organic tin compounds develop symptoms that are very similar to Alzheimer's disease (Corrigan et al. 1991). These similarities heighten speculation as to cause and effect, and underscore the need for further investigation into an area presently lacking in scientific research, particularly given the widespread use of tin cans by the food industry.

CIRCULATORY PROBLEMS OF THE BRAIN

Lack of circulation to the brain has long been suspected as a causative factor of Alzheimer's disease. When blood supply to the brain is decreased, the corresponding supply of oxygen and glucose is reduced, and this can lead to cellular damage and death.

Hardening of the Arteries

Atherosclerotic vascular disease (hardening of the arteries) is now referred to as an Alzheimer's-related disease and has been dismissed as a cause of Alzheimer's. Although controversial, other studies continue to suggest a direct causal link between cerebrovascular disease and Alzheimer's.

Research at the Indiana University School of Medicine revealed how compromised blood flow to the brain could account
for Alzheimer's (Crawford 1996). A German study showed that
ischemia and hypoxia, the respective lack of blood supply and
oxygen to the brain, are causative factors of Alzheimer's (Jendroska et al. 1995). We know that an insufficient supply of blood
and oxygen and inadequate amounts of glucose exact a toll on
brain tissues because they trigger abnormal chemical reactions
that create toxic and excitatory cellular changes. These in turn
result in cellular damage and death with typical Alzheimer's
pathological changes.

TIAs

Of particular interest to researchers are multiple transient ischemic attacks (TIAs)—the "mini-stroke syndrome." The dementia resulting from multiple small strokes is referred to as
"multi-infarct dementia," an Alzheimer-related dementia that
clinically exhibits the same symptoms as Alzheimer's disease. It
reveals a more malignant course than that seen in Alzheimer's,
and the risk of death is double that for men versus women, just
as it is in Alzheimer's (Molsa, Marttila, and Rinne 1995).

Strokes

Once referred to as apoplexy, strokes are now known as CVAs
(cerebrovascular accidents). Unlike the slowly progressing dementia of TIAs, or the even slower dementia seen in hardening
of the arteries (atherosclerosis), CVAs are very sudden. They are

a result of either a blood clot creating a blockage in a larger and more vital artery of the brain than involved in a TIA, or due to a brain hemorrhage. Depending upon which artery and vital area of the brain are involved in a CVA, a related dementia to Alzheimer's can evolve abruptly.

AUTOIMMUNE DISEASE

Antibodies are a major thrust of the immune system, and they defend the body by fighting off foreign invaders such as viruses, bacteria, molds, fungi, and cancer cells. In autoimmune disease the body's own antibodies undergo abnormal changes, mistakenly identifying the body's normal cells as foreign invaders, and they begin to eat up the body's own cells and destroy certain tissues. To understand the possible abnormal autoimmune response that we suspect in Alzheimer's and how normally protective antibodies become harmful agents, we learn from our knowledge of other autoimmune diseases as presented in Exhibit 6.1.

OUR GOAL AND OBJECTIVES

Our goal is to find a complete cure for Alzheimer's. This will be possible when all the underlying causes, pathological changes in the brain, and biochemical reactions leading to these changes are fully understood and totally correctable. We have overcome major hurdles along this path in the past few years and significantly expanded our knowledge of Alzheimer's. Indeed our total world knowledge was doubling every five years in 1970. In 1990, it was doubling at the rate of every five months. It is estimated that to-

---

Exhibit 6.1 Summary of Some Auto-immune Diseases

Rheumatic Fever The beta streptococcal bacteria that cause rheumatic fever are responsible for the proliferation of antibodies that attack the valves of the heart and the joints.

Lupus The antibodies of lupus attack several body tissues, which include the skin, lungs, kidneys, or joints.

Thyroid Disease Antithyroid antibodies slowly destroy thyroid glandular tissues in one type of thyroiditis (inflammation of the thyroid) known as Hashimoto's disease. This causes the thyroid to be replaced eventually by massive scar formations that result in an enlarged, poorly functioning gland known as a goiter.

Brain Antibrain antibodies have been identified against both the central nervous system and a neurotransmitter (Schott et al. 1996). However, this area of study is still in its infancy and the significance of the antibodies is not yet clarified. Another study revealed that an abnormality in B cells, an integral part of our immune system, is created by infection with the Epstein-Barr (mononucleosis) virus. These altered B cells secrete antibodies against the brain's normal amyloid protein, and they are found in higher incidence in Alzheimer's patients, further suggesting an autoimmune role in Alzheimer's disease (Xu and Gaskin 1997).

---

tal world knowledge will double every five weeks in the year 2000. If this rate holds true for Alzheimer's, the future is indeed bright.

Our current objective is the treatment and prevention of Alzheimer's disease. Until recently we were hampered by a serious lack of knowledge of its underlying causes, the internal mechanisms, and destructive brain pathways. Thus, we had no basis for treatment other than superb caregiving. One cannot adequately treat a disease without a proper diagnosis. That capability now exists for Alzheimer's. Understanding the causes and pathogenesis is beginning to reveal a web of treatment options that are very exciting and very effective. Let us recap what we have discussed:

- Knowledge that Alzheimer's can be caused by exposure to heavy metals, certain widely used medications, electromagnetic fields, and prolonged psychological stress will enable us to avoid these exposures.
- Knowledge of the pathogenic pathways such as inflammation, free radical activity, oxidative stress, genetic inheritance, hormonal depletion, amino acid derangement, vitamin deficiency, and electron transport disruption will enable us to counteract these abnormal reactions with specific medications. Some are already in use and showing remarkable results.
- We can now employ readily available corrective measures and prevent progressive brain damage. For example, chronic inflammatory conditions, head trauma, and chronic and recurrent viral infections can now be treated with certain anti-inflammatory agents to slow progression and help prevent Alzheimer's.
- Free radical and oxidative stress damage can be curtailed and prevented by antioxidants such as vitamin E. Other antioxidants are vitamin C, a number of herbs, and proanthocyanidins from pine bark and grapeseed. The combination of antioxidants provide an even stronger response because they are synergistic and potentiate one another.
- There are beneficial overlaps in treatment. Fifteen independent studies show that anti-inflammatory agents act as free radical scavengers and are also effective against oxidative stress damage and cellular death while inhibitory against excitotoxicity damage in the glutamine neurotransmitter pathway (Breitner 1996).

- A damaged electron transport system of mitochondrial DNA can be effectively treated with coenzyme Q10. This supplement enters every cell in the body and significantly helps correct electron transport dysfunction and cellular energy disruption.
- Estrogen, a female hormone and an Alzheimer's preventative, can be replaced postmenopausally by either synthetic prescription drugs or herbal products and certain foods that are very high in phytoestrogen content. It acts as an effective antioxidant and anti-inflammatory.
- Vitamin E, estrogen, H_2 receptor antagonists, and a number of herbs can effectively treat Alzheimer's.

CHAPTER 7

The Genetic Link

GENETIC MUTATION

Familiarization with the terms "chromosome," "gene," "DNA," "mutation," and "allele" are essential to understanding the genetic inheritance of certain subsets of Alzheimer's disease. We will briefly define these terms here.

Chromosomes

Composed of a substance called DNA, each cell in the body holds twenty-three pairs of them. Each chromosome possesses several thousand genes, and all are identical. Chromosomes occur in paired numbers in every cell with the exception of the sperm and egg.

Genes

A short segment of the chromosome itself, all genes contain identical DNA. Not only do genes predetermine the makeup—and characteristics—of every individual, there are over 50,000 of them in every cell in the body. Half of them are inherited from each parent, and they are, in turn, genetically passed on to that individual's children.

DNA

DNA (deoxyribonucleic acid) is a long chainlike structure that is the major component of chromosomes and genes. It is the physical substance of inheritance and is responsible for genetic copying; thus, each succeeding generation is a copy of the previous generation. The characteristics are dependent upon which paired gene from which parent is stronger (dominant) or weaker (recessive).

Mutation

When an embryonic cell continually divides and doubles in size until full growth is achieved, as occurs in its normal growth patterns, an error may occur in the production of its identical copy; remember that each cell's chromosomal and genetic makeups are identical. A mutation is a rare error that occurs in a gene's DNA, and this mutation replicates (repeats the same change) to future generations, thus becoming an inherited mutated gene.

Allele

Genes occur in pairs. One gene of each pair is inherited from the mother, the other from the father, and they are carried in the same location on each paired chromosome. If a mutation causes one gene to create an extra copy of itself, this copy is called an allele. Mutations can be created by both genes in the pair, thus producing two copies, or alleles.

Every protein of the body is controlled by a matched pair of genes. An allele (extra genetic copy of itself) alters the normal makeup of the associated protein in that matched pair of genes, and this mutant allele is in turn inherited by that individual's children, and so forth down the line. This genetic process is responsible for 20 percent of inherited Alzheimer's disease, and this concept provides a very basic understanding of a genetic evolution of Alzheimer's disease.

All mutations and all alleles are not necessarily harmful, however. Some can actually be beneficial.

Suspicion of Inheritance

Several genes responsible for a number of subsets of Alzheimer's disease have now been found, and they are present in a number of different chromosomes. Although the disease is one that is seen normally in the age group of the late sixties and seventies, the majority of cases start at age sixty-five or older. The earlier the onset, the more likely it is caused by a genetic mutation.

THE LATE-ONSET GENES

Maternal Inheritance: The Cytochrome C Oxidase Gene

Children of affected mothers have a significantly higher rate of Alzheimer's than the progeny (offspring) of affected fathers. This is due to a mutation of the DNA of the mitochondria of the cytochrome C oxidase gene (Parker and Davis 1997). The mitochondria function as the cell's engine. The incidence of maternal to paternal linkage is high at 9:1 (Edland et al. 1997), which means that you are nine times more likely to develop Alzheimer's if your mother had it than if your father did.

Chromosome #12

Occurrence of Alzheimer's past age sixty-five is known as "late on-set" and separated into two categories: sporadic and familial. Early-onset Alzheimer's has historically been attributed to genetic mutations and clearly separated from late-onset disease. However, the newest genetic find relates to late-onset Alzheimer's disease, and a gene found on chromosome #12 is believed responsible for possibly 15 percent of all late-onset cases (Pericak-Vance et al. 1997).

Chromosome #19

A gene called apolipoprotein E (APOE) is associated with Alzheimer's and found on chromosome #19. The four different kinds of the APOE gene are referred to as genotypes. For the sake of simplicity we will refer to them E1, E2, E3, and E4.

- Apolipoprotein E1 (APOE 1) is not associated with Alzheimer's, but it is important because it offers protection against coronary disease and heart attacks (Mahieux et al. 1995).
- Apolipoprotein E2 (APOE 2) has been generally accepted as protective and felt to delay the onset of Alzheimer's. But controversy arose about its role when a study performed in Oslo, Norway, showed that APOE 2 allele conferred no protective effects at all. In fact, survival rates of those who carried this allele were found to be significantly lower than the controls (van Duijn et al. 1995). Another study at Duke University concludes with a more optimistic finding that the

presence of APOE 2 allele does not increase early-onset Alzheimer's (Scott et al. 1997). The actual role played by APOE 2 is far too crucial to be left unresolved. Further research may be required to determine its true action and its potential future role in genetic treatment.

- Apolipoprotein E3 (APOE 3) is essentially neutral and has little effect one way or the other on the development of Alzheimer's disease.
- Apolipoprotein E4 (APOE 4) is the harmful gene allele that increases the risk of developing the disease. This mutated gene is responsible for approximately 70 percent of late-onset familial and late-onset sporadic types of Alzheimer's dementia (Roses 1996a; Locke et al. 1995). This increased risk of Alzheimer's is heightened further by secondary associations:

  - If an inherited APOE 4 allele is present in individuals who sustain head trauma, it is responsible for a ten-fold increase of Alzheimer's-type dementia.
  - In patients who suffer from herpes meningitis, a brain infection caused by the herpes simplex virus (HSV 1), APOE 4 is responsible for a much higher incidence of dementia than those who do not harbor this mutant allele.
  - Approximately one-third of Americans have one allele of APOE 4. This puts them at an intermediate risk of genetic determination. Of those who do carry one copy of this gene, estimates are that 90 percent will not develop Alzheimer's, and only 10 percent will.
  - Approximately 2 percent of the population have two copies (alleles) of the APOE 4 gene, which constitutes a far greater risk. This creates a 50 percent chance of

developing Alzheimer's prior to age seventy. Its maximal effects are depleted by age seventy (Blacker et al. 1997).

- The rate of progression of Alzheimer's, however, is independent of APOE 4, although the amount of pathology observed at autopsy may be much greater (Norman et al. 1995).

Apolipoprotein C 1

Another gene called apolipoprotein C 1 has been found close to apolipoprotein E on the same chromosome, #19. It is considered a risk factor for developing Alzheimer's (Podulso et al. 1995).

Chromosomes #4, #6, and #20

New chromosomal sites for mutated genes appear with greater frequency compared to just a few short years ago. Chromosomes presently under investigation for possible genetic links to Alzheimer's are #4, #6, and #20 (Pericak-Vance 1997).

IS GENETIC TESTING FOR APOE 4 RECOMMENDED?

The presence of APOE 4 does not mean that a person will develop Alzheimer's. Testing young people or older individuals who are cognitively intact and without risk factors, purely for predictability, is not warranted or recommended. During a meeting of some of the top scientists in the country in October

1995, it was determined that genetic testing for APOE should be restricted to the use of evaluating confirmed dementia and possibly for selecting therapies (Roses 1996b). Since 90 percent of APOE 4 individuals never develop dementia and 70 percent of the population do not carry APOE 4 at all, the predictive merit of the APOE 4 test is very low, considering its statistical values (Myers et al. 1996).

APOE genotyping (testing) is not sensitive or specific enough to diagnose Alzheimer's disease if used alone as a diagnostic tool; however, its accuracy improves when it is evaluated in combination with clinical evidence (Mayeux et al. 1998).

Nevertheless, there may be important indications for APOE 4 testing. The presence of definite markers or a history of known predisposing circumstances, such as multiple head traumas and recurrent herpes viral meningitis, are carefully selected indications and are shown in Exhibit 7.1.

The markers detailed in Exhibit 7.1 dictate early evaluation. Because Alzheimer's evolves over decades before it becomes perceptually observable, early markers attest to the validity of APOE 4 evaluation as an integral part of the workup, as opposed to unnecessary random testing of the general public. Early diagnosis remains the key to prevention

To summarize, APOE 4 denotes late-onset dementia at age sixty-five and older, of both sporadic and familial types, for which a mutated gene on chromosome #19 may be responsible. A mutant gene is also present on chromosome #12, which is now believed responsible for 15 percent of late-onset cases. Hereditary mutations found in chromosomal locations different from the mutation of chromosome #12, or the mutant APOE 4 allele on chromosome #19, are responsible for early-onset Alzheimer's, spanning age thirty through age sixty-five. If there is a def-

---

Exhibit 7.1 Nine Unusual Situations for Which Genetic Testing for APOE 4 Is Advised

1. *Fingerprint patterns* are a marker that can predict the development of Alzheimer's years prior to its onset, thus negating the recommendation to wait for the disease to evolve clinically before testing.

2. *A clear family history* of multiple cases, particularly on the maternal side and spanning generations, is another definite marker and indication for testing.

3. *Recurring herpes viral meningitis* can be a dangerous precursor if the individual is a carrier of APOE 4. In these cases, testing is mandatory.

4. *Recurrent head trauma* is of particular significance when loss of consciousness is involved since there is a tenfold increase of developing Alzheimer's when the individual is a carrier of the APOE 4 gene.

5. *Recent memory loss* is a very early objective symptom. Early memory loss justifies APOE 4 testing as part of testing to confirm the disease.

6. *Loss of the sensation of smell* is a very early symptom and reliable marker, giving caretakers up to two years' warning. It justifies immediate testing as opposed to waiting for the disease to evolve. Early diagnosis augments early treatment and may lead to prevention.

7. *Visuospatial disturbance* occurs early and is easily tested at home by the "clock test" or professionally by the Benton Visual Retention Test.

8. *Hearing loss* is a very early symptom with a very high percentage of occurrence.

9. *Onset of depression* among sixty- or seventy-year-olds with no prior history of depression and no apparent recent cause is a situation in which testing is advisable.

---

inite diagnosis of early-onset or a family history of early-onset along with early short-term memory loss in the patient, then genetic testing should be directed instead to those mutated genes responsible for early-onset Alzheimer's.

In particular, there are specific mutations present on chromosomes numbered 1, 14, and 21 that cause early-onset disease (Roses 1997).

THE EARLY-ONSET GENES

Chromosome #14

There are two closely related mutated genes which have been identified, called the presenilins One of these genes, presenilin #1, is found on chromosome #14. Presenilin #1 accounts for 70 percent of patients with early-onset Alzheimer's disease and surfaces between ages thirty and sixty-five. A group of scientists in Belgium found forty-two distinct mutations on the presenilin #1 gene (Cruts and Van Broeckhoven 1998).

Chromosome #1

The second related gene, presenilin #2, is found on chromosome #1, and it is responsible for 25 percent of patients with early-onset Alzheimer's disease. Two actual mutations have been found on this gene (Cruts, Hendricks, and Van Broekhoven 1996).

Presenilins and Oxidative Stress

Presenilin-mutated genes create an oxidative stress reaction in the brain with an outpouring of calcium from affected brain cells. This abnormal chain of events disrupts the mitochondria and electron transfer (the cell's energy) and results in nerve degeneration and death (Guo et al. 1997). It is felt that antioxidants such as vitamin E and calcium channel blockers, a prescription medicine used mainly to treat high blood pressure and angina (heart pain), are effective agents in counteracting these adverse genetic effects and thus slowing the progression of the disease.

Early Seizures

Unexplained seizures may spell an early marker for this rare but severe subset of early Alzheimer's (Campion et al. 1996). Research in France identified a single family whose affected members ranged in age from twenty-nine to thirty-five when the diagnoses were made. Two members of this family suffered from seizures. The initial presenting symptoms were those of marked muscle and limb spasticity and epileptic-type seizures that occurred several years prior to the onset of dementia.

Chromosome #21

The remaining 5 percent of early-onset cases are due to a genetic mutation on chromosome #21. The combination of all three gene mutations accounts for early-onset disease, with the youngest case on record at age twenty-nine.

The mutated gene on chromosome #21 is known as the amyloid precursor protein (APP) gene. This mutant is responsible for approximately 5 percent of familial Alzheimer's disease of early onset (Schellenberg 1995). Amyloid is a normal brain protein. It becomes toxic through one of many mechanisms, including its own mutagenic actions, and it becomes embodied in plaque (clump) formations between brain cells. Normal amyloid protein is thus the precursor of abnormal plaquing since it can become toxic and form clumps on the RASP receptors of nerve cells. APP is believed to act as a common pathway for the development of Alzheimer's. A mutant gene found on chromosome #21 controls this protein precursor's progress into that of toxic plaque (Lendon, Ashall, and Goate 1997; Sandbrink et al. 1996). When

Table 7.1 Summary of Genetic Risks

Maternal Inheritance	Caused by the cytochrome oxidase gene. Mother's linkage is greater than linkage through the father by 9:1.

The Late-Onset Genes

Chromosome #12	Responsible for 15 percent of late-onset cases.
Chromosome #19	Contains the APOE 4 (apolipoprotein E 4) allele, responsible for late-onset sporadic and familial cases and causes greater risk with head trauma, herpes simplex 1 viral meningitis (brain) infection, recent memory loss, and a positive family history.
Apolipoprotein C 1	Found close to apolipoprotein E on the same chromosome, #19. Considered a risk factor for developing Alzheimer's.

The Early-Onset Genes: 15–20 percent of inherited cases

Chromosome #14	Carries the presenilin #1 gene. Responsible for 70 percent of early-onset cases.
Chromosome #1	Carries the presenilin #2 gene. Responsible for 25 percent of early-onset cases.
Chromosome #21	Carries the amyloid precursor protein (APP) gene. Responsible for 5 percent of early-onset cases. Causes protein to clump out in the brain. Decreased levels of APP in cerebrospinal fluid act as a marker for the disease.
HLA 2A Gene	Carriers develop the disease two to four years earlier than Alzheimer's patients who do not possess the allele.
Chromosomes #4, #6, and #20	Chromosomes presently under investigation for possible genetic links to Alzheimer's.

APP clumps in the brain, its level in the cerebrospinal fluid lowers. Decreasing levels of APP fragments correspond to decreasing degrees of cognition. Measurement of this fragment of APP in the cerebrospinal fluid is used as a marker to diagnose Alzheimer's disease.

HLA-2A Gene

Alzheimer's patients who carry the HLA-2A gene, or a closely linked gene, are found to develop the disease two to four years earlier than Alzheimer's patients who do not possess it. Since it may play a role in the inflammatory process, it might be responsive to anti-inflammatories (Small et al. 1997).

GENETIC IMMUNITY

Just as there are families and groups who show a higher incidence of inheritance (genetic predisposition) to developing Alzheimer's, there are groups who exhibit immunity such as the Cherokee Nation of Native Americans. Studies at the University of Texas indicate increased immunity with increased ancestry, which has been clearly protective. This protection decreases as ancestry diminishes by dilution with marriage into nontribal populations (Rosenberg et al. 1996).

A study in France revealed that moderate daily wine consumption imparts some degree of immunity against Alzheimer's disease (Orgogozo et al. 1997). Of the individuals studied, 250 to 500 ml of wine daily was considered moderate. However, genetic predisposition was not a factor in this study.

CHAPTER 8

Testing

There are numerous tests currently available that are able to differentiate Alzheimer's from many other types of related dementias. As stated so many times thus far, Alzheimer's has historically been a diagnosis of exclusion with autopsy as the sole method of definitive diagnosis. Because of overlapping symptoms, however, other dementias and disease states must first be ruled out.

PROFESSIONAL EVALUATION

All testing begins with a thorough evaluation by the family practitioner, internist, or gerontologist, and a neurologist or psychiatrist may be consulted.

LITTLE-KNOWN MARKERS:
"DO-IT-YOURSELF" HOME TESTING

Abnormalities occur in Alzheimer's long before the disease presents itself. These are markers, very early warning signs, and indicate that something may be wrong with further evaluation warranted. A few of these markers can be confirmed with keen observation at home.

Fingerprint Patterns

Fingerprint patterns provide an early marker in identifying Alzheimer's years before its onset. Typically, radial loops (normal fingerprint loops) point toward the thumb and are found mainly on the index and large fingers. Others loops may point straight toward the end of the digit, neither toward nor away from the thumb and are of no clinical importance. Of greatest clinical significance are ulnar loops that point away from the thumb, toward the little finger, and it is their abnormal presence that indicates early Alzheimer's. Other fingerprint structures known as whorls and arches may be seen (Figure 8.1). Patterns are simple to detect with a light source held at an angle, such as from a penlight type of flashlight and a magnifying glass. It is a relatively accurate test and an extremely early marker for the disease.

Pattern Changes Found in Alzheimer's
In Alzheimer's disease, there are revealing pattern changes:

1. There is a significant increase in the ulnar loops (pointing away from the thumb). This is crucial in very early diagnosis. Eight or more ulnar loops are found in 72 percent of Alzheimer's patients' fingertips, while only 26 percent of the normal control group show this pattern, thus raising a red flag possibly years before symptoms arise.
2. A decrease in whorls and arches occurs in Alzheimer's, but they increase in other dementias.
3. The radial loops (pointing toward the thumb), if present at all, and normally found on the index and large

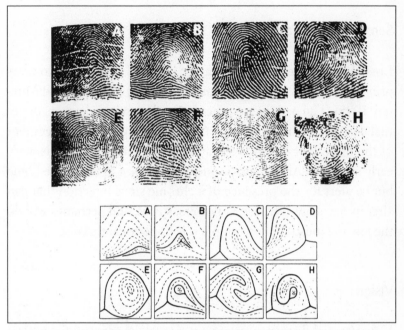

Figure 8.1 Types of fingerprint patterns. *Top*: Actual prints. *Bottom*: Schematic drawings with pattern-type lines. *A* indicates simple arch; *B*, tented arch; *C*, ulnar loop; *D*, radial loop; *E*, simple whorl; *F*, central-pocket whorl; *G*, double-loop whorl; and *H*, accidental whorl.

fingers, are now shifted to the ring and little fingers (Weinrob 1985).

The same patterns are found in Down's syndrome. In fact, all Down's syndrome patients will develop Alzheimer's disease if they survive past age forty. The abnormal genes for both Alzheimer's and Down's syndrome are found on the same chromosome, #19. Genetic testing is very strongly recommended if your patterns are a positive match; if there is an associated family history of Alzheimer's, genetic testing is imperative.

Sense-of-Smell Test

Loss of the sensation of smell can be detected as early as two years prior to onset of cognitive symptoms (Morgan, Nordin, and Murphy 1995). The pathogenesis lies in the disruption, damage, or actual destruction of nerve cells in the olfactory lobe (that segment of the brain that controls the ability to detect odors). This very early marker of Alzheimer's is one of the easiest to test in the home but be alert for the presence of a chronic sinus infection that can alter its accuracy. The use of flowers, spices, and perfumes will do the job and illustrate how simple it is to perform this test.

Vision

Visual/spatial disturbances are a very early marker of disease but should be evaluated by a professional. If a home test is all that is possible, however, do the following. Have the person observe ten items laid out on a tablecloth for one minute. Tell the person to look away and then ask for a "recall" of the items and their positions to one another. Have other family members do the same test. Compare the family's results. If the suspected person's score is very low, that is suggestive of Alzheimer's.

A very popular and simple test for visual/spatial assessment is the "clock test." The person with suspected Alzheimer's is asked to look at a clock, observe the position of its hands, and then look away and draw what was observed. Alzheimer's is suspected if the individual has difficulty reproducing what was seen and draws all the numbers to one side or places the clock's hands in the wrong position.

Hearing

Hearing loss is a very early and prevalent marker, occurring long before objective symptoms appear. The patient is generally not aware of any hearing loss.

Accurate testing is normally best done by a professional according to established protocol, but minimal observation at home can provide an accurate assessment. Does someone need to raise a voice before the patient will hear it? Is the television constantly turned up loud? Do you have to repeat things? Are you constantly misunderstood? Does it appear that someone is not paying attention or even listening to you? Even though hearing loss may be due to an old injury, chronic disease, impacted cerumen (wax), or vascular disease, it is so much more prevalent in Alzheimer's than in any other disease state that it is a reliable marker.

Depression

Depression is a psychiatric disorder that can surface more than two years before the onset of cognitive symptoms of Alzheimer's. There are subtle changes in both behavior and mood long before the onset of perceptual symptoms: poor appetite, social withdrawal, a desire to be left alone, a prolonged period of tiredness, decreased affect, no interest, no goals, crying spells, and no desire to go anywhere or do anything.

When these symptoms begin without any obvious reason for depression such as the death of a loved one, an acute or chronic illness, or financial burdens, then it should be suspected as a pre-Alzheimer's dementia.

NEUROPSYCHOLOGICAL TESTING

There are many neuropsychological tests with specific areas of testing and comparative values. Single tests such as those for vision or speech only are popular. There are test batteries, combinations of single tests covering such abilities as cognition, behavior, speech, visual spacial perceptions, manual dexterity, and attention.

An outstanding test battery is the Standardized Alzheimer's Disease Assessment Scale (SADAS), covering all areas of major importance (Standish et al. 1996).

Researchers at the National Institute on Aging utilized the Benton Visual Retention Test (BVRT) and were able to predict the onset of Alzheimer's prior to the onset of cognitive symptoms. This test can be used as an early marker because of its superior accuracy and early results.

An interesting comparison of test batteries versus single tests was done at the University of Toronto. A simple subset of the popular Wechsler Memory Scale and a delayed recall from the Rey Auditory Verbal Learning Test were compared with larger test batteries and resulted in the same accuracy as their larger-scale models. These results concluded that relatively brief testing can be exceptionally accurate (Tierney et al. 1996). This is akin to predicting the national elections with 3 to 5 percent of the vote reporting.

In another study, a comparison of five neuropsychological tests of Alzheimer's revealed equal and sometimes better accuracy with shorter, rather than longer, testing procedures (Stuss et al. 1996). Single category tests or simple abbreviated tests that provide proven comparable results to more intricate tests and test batteries are obviously easier for the patient to take and more cost effective as well.

"The 7-Minute Screen," a test with a reported accuracy of 92 percent, is currently under evaluation. Developed by Dr. P. R. Solomon at Williams College, Williamstown, Massachusetts, it encompasses intellectual functioning and is reportedly able to differentiate between Alzheimer's and senility. Hopefully, this test will prove itself accurate and be available soon for simple, rapid testing in every physician's office.

A test developed at Columbia University accurately predicts the time remaining until the patient requires placement in a nursing facility prior to death. It is based on cognitive test scores and described in the literature as very accurate. It's the first of its kind and, hopefully, will be available soon (Stern et al. 1997).

There are numerous neuropsychological tests in routine use, many of which are excellent. Although it is not within the scope of this book to describe all of them, a few are noted to give the reader a more complete understanding of the many evaluative tests.

CEREBROSPINAL FLUID PROTEINS

In describing the accuracy of testing such as cerebrospinal fluid and scanning (imaging) procedures, reference is made throughout the book to specificity and sensitivity.

- *Specificity* is the ability of a test to clearly distinguish a given (specific) disease from other diseases: to clearly isolate it.
- *Sensitivity* refers to the degree (percent) of accuracy with which a test can diagnose that particular disease.

The cerebrospinal fluid is the milieu (or fluid medium) that bathes the inside of the brain and spinal cord. The proteins and chemicals within this fluid reflect the metabolic functions of the brain. When certain abnormalities such as Alzheimer's disease and many of its related dementias affect the brain, these diseases may be telegraphed by an increase or decrease in the amounts of specific proteins in the cerebrospinal fluid. The abnormal presence or amounts of these proteins can often be used as markers or as diagnostic tests to indicate pathological changes occurring in the brain. The recent discovery of these proteins represents a monumental breakthrough in the diagnosis of Alzheimer's, incorporated into highly accurate markers and tests that are already in clinical use with others still in the investigational stage.

AD 7 C

The most significant cerebrospinal fluid test to date is called AD 7 C. Its sensitivity is approximately 90 percent, and it approaches autopsy for accuracy (de la Monte et al. 1996). AD 7 C tests for a particular protein called the neural thread protein, which is detected at ten times greater in Alzheimer's patients than in normal counterpart controls. It elevates early in the course of the disease, and it increases as the disease progresses. Research indicates that this protein evolves from nerve cells in the brain, and it is involved with their repair and regeneration. While the other cerebrospinal tests in current use are considered markers, AD 7 C is diagnostic.

It is also being released to the marketplace as a simple urine test to be available in every physician's office, thus avoiding the rigors of a spinal tap. Both the time and costs involved to diagnose Alzheimer's with superior accuracy by merely dropping off a urine specimen are drastically reduced, and the answer is available within forty-eight hours instead of after weeks or months of scheduling appointments, interviews, multiple tests, and procedures. This represents a potential major breakthrough in early diagnosis of Alzheimer's.

Amyloid Precursor Protein (APP)

Amyloid precursor protein (APP) is a fragment of normal amyloid protein of the brain that has become toxic. This reaction is predetermined by an inherited mutated gene found on chromosome #21 and is responsible for 5 percent of early-onset cases. When this protein fragment becomes toxic, it clumps out in the brain and its levels become decreased in the cerebrospinal fluid. By measuring this lowered protein level, we are thereby able to use the test as a marker for the disease. The lower the level drops, the poorer the performance reflected in attention, recent memory, intelligence, and other cognitive abilities. Because there is overlap of results with diseases other than Alzheimer's, its sensitivity is reduced to approximately 25 percent, thus relegating it to a marker rather than a diagnostic test.

Tau Protein

Tau, another abnormal protein found in the cerebrospinal fluid, is produced by the degradation of nerve cells and is present in significantly greater amounts early in Alzheimer's. The greater the degree of dementia, the higher the level of tau. Because it

Table 8.1 Comparison of AD 7 C, APP, and Tau

	Sensitivity	Overlap
	Percent of Alzheimer's Cases Detected	Percent of Alzheimer's and Normals in the Same Range
AD 7 C	80–90	5–7
APP	25	80–85
Tau	25	80–90

Source: Taken from physician information release produced by Nymox Pharmaceutical Corporation.

reaches critical levels early, it is an excellent marker for early detection of disease. CSF tau concentration is substantially increased compared with controls in mild Alzheimer's disease and in other forms of dementia, suggesting that raised tau concentration is a nonspecific marker of neuronal degeneration (Riemenschneider et al. 1997). Although its specificity for identifying Alzheimer's is only 50 percent, there is overlap with other dementias, reducing its sensitivity to 25 percent (Riemenschneider et al. 1997). For a comparison of the AD 7 C, APP, and Tau tests, see Table 8.1.

Synaptotagmin

Synaptotagmin is present in both the brain and cerebrospinal fluid. Studies at the University of Göteborg in Sweden show a marked reduction of this protein both in the cerebrospinal fluid and in brain tissue, particularly the hippocampus, with early onset Alzheimer's disease (Davidsson et al. 1996). Although still too early to qualify as a marker or diagnostic test, it shows exceptional promise.

AMY 117

This newly discovered protein, found only in Alzheimer's patients, is abundant in the brain and found in plaquelike protein lesions. It has the potential to evolve more as a diagnostic marker for Alzheimer's than the toxic amyloid protein plaques (APP) (Trojanowski 1997).

AST

AST (aspartate aminotransferase) is a molecule produced by impaired glucose metabolism. In comparative studies with other dementias, it was found that AST is specific for Alzheimer's and not present in other dementias tested, nor in the control group. This makes AST a potential marker for differentiating Alzheimer's from other dementias. When the results of AST are evaluated along with those of tau, the specificity (specific accuracy for a single disease) of tau improves from 50 to 83 percent (Riemenschneider et al. 1997).

IMAGING

There are several types of imaging modalities that are utilized for both diagnostic and therapeutic purposes. The PET scan is better for the diagnosis of Alzheimer's; the CAT scan is better for the diagnosis of non-Alzheimer's disease states. MRI and SPECT scans have been utilized in part to diagnose Alzheimer's and exclude related dementias.

PET Scan

The PET scan (positron emission tomography) is the most advanced imaging technique known to medical science today. It measures blood flow, glucose utilization, oxygen consumption, and metabolism in the brain. Instead of using X rays or magnetism, or protons, the PET scan emits positron rays that significantly increase its capabilities.

This makes it capable of multiple functions regarding the Alzheimer's process:

- can significantly aid in diagnosis
- can monitor the disease's development and progression
- can check the effects of new therapies used in treatment

Use of the newer three-dimensional PET scan gives it the marked ability to diagnose Alzheimer's with an accuracy of 94 percent sensitivity and 99 percent specificity. Its accuracy is exceptional in mild dementia as well as in very early cases where only clinical suspicion exists (Reiman et al. 1996; Burdette et al. 1996).

The 3-D PET scan is evolving into the most accurate diagnostic tool yet devised. It has the potential of becoming *the* primary diagnostic tool in Alzheimer's disease. It is speculated that 3-D PET scans will eventually be able to predict the onset of Alzheimer's twenty years prior to onset by detecting obscure changes in brain metabolism. Unfortunately, its high cost and sparse availability severely limit its present use. There are only a limited number of 3-D PET scanners throughout the United States, with the vast majority found at major universities. A percentage of their use is restricted to research studies. Eventually, its cost will drop substantially, its availability will markedly improve, and its predictive accuracy will advance as did the X ray, CAT scanner, and MRI.

SPECT Scan

The SPECT scan (single photon emission computed tomography) is another imaging technique, but its precision in diagnosing Alzheimer's is not as good as other methods, and it does not contribute substantially to an accurate diagnosis. Its specificity is 89 percent, and its sensitivity is only 43 percent (Van Gool 1995). However, the newer three-dimensional SPECT scan is more accurate than the Single Photon Emission Scan (Bergman et al. 1997), and it does provide a higher degree of diagnostic accuracy from Alzheimer's when utilized with a perfusion test showing a portion of the brain known as the temporoparietal area. A perfusion test measures how rapidly or effectively blood passes through (perfuses) the particular tissue being examined. A SPECT perfusion test shows clearly on film the actual flow of blood into brain tissues. Defects and abnormal structural changes shown in the perfusion of this particular brain segment indicate a 95 percent sensitivity for Alzheimer's and a specificity of 60 percent. This is far better than the plain single emission scan (Ishii et al. 1996). It is not able to measure glucose uptake or brain metabolism that catapults the PET scan to the acme of imaging.

CAT Scan

The CAT scan (computed axial tomography) is most effective when imaging bone for problems such as undetectable hairline fractures, arthritis, and the spread of cancer. As a tool for evaluation of the brain and dementias, however, it is more accurate for diagnosing circulatory disease and strokes than for diagnosing Alzheimer's (Lopez et al. 1995).

MRI

The classical MRI finding in Alzheimer's is the clear distinction of both hippocampal and temporal lobe atrophy (Xanthakos et al. 1996). Hippocampal atrophy can be recognized by volumetric measurement with an MRI even before the appearance of symptoms surfaces (Fox et al. 1996).

Alzheimer's symptoms usually don't present until billions of nerve cells are destroyed. The advent of the 3-D MRI has greatly enhanced diagnosis and the ability to monitor the progression of Alzheimer's. It is 95 percent accurate.

The MRI (magnetic resonance imaging) avoids X rays and uses magnetism. It shows soft tissues such as the brain and spinal cord far better than a CAT scan, and it shows the hippocampal brain segment quite well also (an area that atrophies up to 8 percent per year in Alzheimer's). It also shows the temporal lobes very well, a diagnostic necessity because this area is entrenched in the Alzheimer's process. The downhill progression of disease can be closely monitored using an MRI (Fox et al. 1996). Atrophy is also denoted in other areas of the brain.

EEG

The EEG (electroencephalogram) tests brain wave patterns. Although it is an aid in diagnosis, it is not specific to Alzheimer's because brain waves show slowing in other disease states as well as Alzheimer's. This creates a lowered specificity and reliability for this type of test.

BEAM

The BEAM, (brain electrical activity mapping) test evaluates the velocity of brain waves. A slow speed reflects a high risk factor for Alzheimer's. Specificity is not optimal in this test because velocity is also slowed in other disease states such as anxiety, depression, abuse of alcohol and cocaine, and Parkinson's disease (Braverman et al. 1997a; Braverman et al. 1997b).

BLOOD TESTING

A complete battery of tests is required to rule out many disease states that mimic the symptoms of Alzheimer's dementia and cloud the diagnosis. These include a CBC, SMA panel, serology, HIV 1, ANA, drugs (prescription and illicit), heavy metals, B_{12} and folate levels, hormone levels, thyroid, and urinalysis. An APOE 4 may be indicated as part of the clinical workup. Although these abbreviations may be unfamiliar to you, they are employed to separate out many diseases with symptoms that overlap those of Alzheimer's.

A confirmed diagnosis of Alzheimer's does not automatically rule out other underlying related dementias. For example, suppose both a PET scan and an AD 7 C cerebrospinal test were positive for Alzheimer's: it would indeed provide a diagnosis as accurate as autopsy. However, what guarantee would we have that the patient's proven Alzheimer's disease was not combined with a related dementia such as one created by an underactive thyroid, frontotemporal dementia, or pernicious anemia? If this were the case, which dementia would present the greater problem? How many other disease states would require treatment? Fifteen percent of dementias are Alzheimer's-related, and 15 percent are mixed. We must still rule out other potentially related dementias in order to institute appropriate treatment.

Ultimately, we must rely on the physician's clinical experience in interpreting results from blood and cerebrospinal fluid testing, scanning procedures, cognition testing, and motor and sensory testing in order to arrive at a correct diagnosis.

OTHER TESTS

There have been several studies using the eye drop tropicamide for pupil dilation. It measures the integrity of the cholinergic neurotransmitter pathway by evaluating the change in pupil size. The pupil dilates when a drop is applied. Although designed as a test for Alzheimer's, other neurological diseases that also involve the brain's cholinergic neurotransmitters mar the results because specificity is poor. Thus, it is not the most ideal of tests. A study on an Alzheimer's group from the Mayo Clinic, in fact, showed no evidence that tropicamide possesses any efficacy as a diagnostic test (FitzSimon et al. 1997).

CHAPTER 9

Research

We cannot begin to equate the financial costs of Alzheimer's to the suffering experienced by its 4 million victims, or the pain, agony, and frustration of the 20 million Americans directly affected by this disease. Although 4 million have been diagnosed, another 4 million or more are already in the preclinical stages without a clue as to what awaits them.

FUNDING

Funding in this country is threefold. The U.S. government provides over $350 million per year toward research. Given that Alzheimer's is the fourth leading cause of death in the United States at a cost of over $100 billion per year for diagnosis, treatment, medications, doctors' fees, and hospital and nursing home expenses, $350 million worth of research pales in light of these expenses and the concomitant suffering. It is estimated that national expenditures can be pared to $50 billion just by slowing the course of this disease.

Statistically, one in every nine women will have breast cancer and one in every seven men will have prostate cancer, but one in every two Americans will eventually develop Alzheimer's disease if they live to age eighty-five. An aging uncle once advised me as a very young boy: "What I was, you are. What I am, you will be!" What are our chances really like?

None of these statistics is acceptable, of course, especially a 50 percent Alzheimer's expectancy rate. Greater funding is paramount. We took the bull by the horns in the past and wiped out a host of diseases including yellow fever, smallpox, polio, diphtheria, and measles. With the same concerted effort and appropriate funding, I have no doubt that Alzheimer's will one day be a disease of the past. I am confident that we can find a cure.

The second major source of funding is from international pharmaceutical companies. This money goes directly into research and development, a $359 million investment per drug. Two drugs have been approved for the treatment of Alzheimer's disease, and of the 3,000 drugs currently in various stages of development, over 100 are being researched as Alzheimer's treatments. However, it takes twelve to fifteen years before the FDA grants final approval to market a single drug. As a result, tremendous costs are unavoidable due to high research and development expenses, meeting prudent FDA safety regulations, and high-end promotion once a drug has received approval.

The third source of funding is the nonprofit Alzheimer's Association and the many beautiful people who support it. In my mind, it represents the most admirable and commendable source of funding for research. Private funding accounts for greater than $50 million annually, the result of an impressive effort by caring and loving individuals.

DIRECTIONS OF DRUG RESEARCH

Research must be directed against the underlying causes, pathogenesis, physiological, and biochemical interactions of disease. Different drugs are being directed toward different metabolic actions. The publication "Investigational Drugs Quarterly" lists over 3,000 investigational drugs either applied for or in initial application, experimental research, preclinical stage, or phases I, II, and III of clinical trials. Here are some of the basic areas of drug research directed against Alzheimer's.

1. *The acetylcholine (cholinergic) neurotransmitter system.* For improvement in memory and attention, it is essential to increase the available neurotransmitter, acetylcholine. To accomplish this, efforts to reduce anticholinesterase, a type of check-and-balance enzyme responsible for lowering acetylcholine levels, is presently a favorite strategy in research. Cognex and Aricept, two drugs already approved by the FDA, both belong to this family of anticholinesterase enzyme inhibitors.

2. *The glutamine neurotransmitter system.* Efforts are being made to prevent excitotoxic changes that cause nerve damage and death in this neurotransmitter system. Anti-inflammatory medications such as vitamin E, ibuprofen, and H_2 blockers such as Tagamet are currently the agents of choice to block excitotoxic cell death.

3. *Amyloid plaquing.* Research is focusing on preventing the formation of toxic plaques between brain cells that result in neuronal death. Agents are presently under study that have been shown to prevent plaque stickiness and adherence.

4. *Hormonal etiologies.* We know about the role of decreasing hormone levels such as estrogen, melatonin, and DHEA in the aging body. As indicated previously,

melatonin helps regulate circadian (day-night) rhythms
and is a free radical scavenger, while DHEA exists at
levels 48 percent lower in Alzheimer's patients compared to their normal counterparts, and may have a
potential role in the treatment of the disease.

5. *Stimulation of nerve cells.* A substance called nerve
growth factor (NGF) that promotes nerve growth and
protects, repairs, and regenerates nerve cells is under
study. After a loss of up to one-third of these nerve
cells in experimental rats, NGF was shown to restore
cognition to normal. Human trials are now in their
second phase and hold promise of producing a dramatic breakthrough.

6. *Anti-inflammatory agents.* Aimed at underlying inflammatory brain changes, these agents are already providing effective prevention.

7. *Antioxidants.* Research has proven them essential and
effective in the prevention of free radical damage and
oxidative stress. They are already proven in the treatment and prevention of Alzheimer's and heart disease.

8. *Genetic therapy.* Although several mutant genes have
been identified, more are yet to be found through genetic research. Identification is not enough; mutations
must be corrected.

9. *Electromagnetism.* Though in its infancy, research
strongly implicates it as a cause of Alzheimer's.

10. *Over-the-counter medications and prescription drugs.* The
prolonged use of several medicines such as chlorpromazine are emerging with negative ramifications toward Alzheimer's. Other medicines have proven

themselves significantly beneficial in a protective role such as estrogen, ibuprofen (Motrin), nicotine, vitamin E, and coenzyme Q10.

11. *Diet and proper food consumption: Proper nutrients.* This has long been a neglected area of research and treatment. Fatty foods and excessive calorie consumption increase oxidative stress and inflammation. In turn, these promote mitochondrial damage and cellular death. Consumption of fish delays Alzheimer's because it provides omega-3 oil, the "good fat."

12. *Electron transport.* Protection of the mitochondria from damage and disruption of the production and transport of energy is an essential part of any treatment and prevention plan. Electron transport needs to be enhanced to prevent harmful brain changes.

CURRENTLY AVAILABLE MEDICINES THAT ARE WELL RESEARCHED AND EFFECTIVE

There are a number of clinically proven and highly effective medications, both over-the-counter and by prescription, that are utilized worldwide for the treatment of Alzheimer's disease. They include vitamins, minerals, and herbal formulas. Some are useful only to treat symptoms, while others show ability to retard and prevent progression of disease. Only those agents that are FDA-approved and clinically effective are recommended here in the treatment plan for Alzheimer's.

The following have been proven effective in the prevention of Alzheimer's disease.

Anti-Inflammatory Agents (Over-the-Counter)

Nearly all research on anti-inflammatories for treatment of Alzheimer's has utilized ibuprofen, but other agents, previously by prescription only, such as the generics for Naprosyn and Orudis, are now readily available. They provide up to 60 percent protection against developing Alzheimer's as determined in a fourteen-year study of over 2,000 older persons conducted at Johns Hopkins School of Public Health (Stewart et al. 1997). Aspirin and acetaminophen (Tylenol) are not effective, however.

A Canadian study reveals a probable effective role for anti-inflammatories against several types of cells seen in suspected autodestructive processes found in Alzheimer's. These findings are a culmination of two separate studies in 1995 and 1996. In the initial study, Indocin, a powerful anti-inflammatory, stopped the progression of the disease (McGeer and McGeer 1996).

An earlier study at Johns Hopkins Alzheimer's Disease Research Center confirms the efficacy of anti-inflammatories and the failure of aspirin and Tylenol (Rich et al. 1995).

A study at Duke University showed there are two separate inflammatory reactions that occur in the brain. both types respond to treatment by NSAIDs (nonsteroidal anti-inflammatories) such as Motrin (ibuprofen). The anti-inflammatories block excitotoxic cell death induced by H_2-type histamine as well as the excitotoxic cell death seen in cells whose synapses are dependent on calcium (Breitner et al. 1996).

Very strong anti-inflammatory and immunosuppressive drugs used in the treatment of some cancers produce maintained improvement of Alzheimer's dementia (Keimowitz 1997).

Estrogen (Prescription Only)

A breakthrough study at the Johns Hopkins Alzheimer's Disease Research Center reveals that estrogen reduces the risk of Alzheimer's by 55 percent. Of major significance, it shows estrogen to be an antioxidant, an anti-inflammatory, and an enhancer of the growth of producing acetylcholine neurons (Kawas et al. 1997). One study at Columbia University showed a decreased risk of Alzheimer's of 40 percent due to taking estrogen for ten years following menopause. A significant study at the University of Southern California showed that the risk of Alzheimer's decreased with increased duration of estrogen replacement (Paganini-Hill and Henderson 1996).

Research at USC also revealed improved cognitive skills in Alzheimer's women given estrogen replacement (Henderson, Watt, and Buckwalter 1996). Both cognition and mood were found to be improved with estrogen supplementation (Chakravorty and Halbreich 1997). Depression is a major problem, since 50 percent of all Alzheimer's patients suffer from it. We know that blocking reuptake of the neurotransmitter serotonin by medications such as Prozac or herbs such as St. John's wort is very effective in treating depression. Estrogen replacement therapy has also been found effective in blunting depression because it adds to the effectiveness of these antidepressants (Halbreich et al. 1995). Thus, these studies unquestionably reflect a direct correlation in women suffering from Alzheimer's and postmenopausal estrogen deficiency.

Estrogen has been found to possess anti-inflammatory and antioxidant properties, too. It promotes the growth of nerve cells that produce the neurotransmitter acetylcholine and improves cognitive skills in Alzheimer's women. It retards the progression of Alzheimer's. Based on a sixteen-year investigation known as the Baltimore Longitudinal Study on Aging (BLSA), participants were tested separately with anti-inflammatories (NSAIDs) and estrogen. In both groups, Alzheimer's was reduced equally by 55 percent (Stewart et al. 1996). It is therefore important that women start estrogen during the perimenopausal time period when symptoms of menopause begin. If there is a personal or strong family history of breast cancer, a woman and her physician may decide that she is not a candidate for estrogen replacement therapy (ERT). Unless there are contraindications to taking estrogen, no postmenopausal woman should be without it.

To summarize the wide range of benefits, estrogen:

- prevents osteoporosis
- prevents heart attacks by 40 to 50 percent
- lowers cholesterol by approximately 10 percent
- functions as an antioxidant
- functions as an anti-inflammatory
- functions as an immune booster
- promotes growth of acetylcholine-producing nerve cells
- improves cognitive skills in Alzheimer's women
- improves mood
- assists in blunting depression
- slows skin wrinkling
- increases blood levels of superoxide desmutase, a very powerful antioxidant
- is assisted by estrogen receptor sites within the coronary arteries
- reduces the chances for Alzheimer's by 55 percent

Although controversy exists in studies correlating estrogen therapy with breast cancer, a review of twenty-seven studies of birth control pills and sixteen studies of postmenopausal estrogen replacement therapy reveals that neither poses any significant effect on the risk of breast cancer (Khoo and Chick 1992).

Nevertheless, for those women with contraindications against estrogen such as family or personal history of breast cancer, fibrocystic breast disease, abnormal or postmenopausal bleeding, endometriosis, fear of estrogen, or because your physician restricts it, there is another option that is as effective and even safer than synthetic estrogen. Phytoestrogens, which are natural plant estrogens and are found in foodstuffs, not only provide the same clinical benefits as synthetic prescriptions, they also significantly decrease the chances of developing cancers—breast cancer in particular. There are numerous studies that conclusively support this finding. Soy, in particular, is very high in phytoestrogens, and one cup of soybeans per day supplies the same amount of estrogen as one tablet of the synthetic estrogen Premarin.

What about the effect of estrogen on the male gender? We don't know yet. There has been a nonfeminizing form of estrogen released to the marketplace, and several others are in the pipeline at present. It may take years to learn what effects they might have on preventing Alzheimer's in men.

Nicotine (Prescription and Over-the-Counter)

Nicotine slows the progression of Alzheimer's. Specialized cells known as nicotinic receptors are located in the synapses and improve learning and memory, an action that is achieved by cholinergic enhancement (Whitehouse and Kalaria 1995). This is accomplished with a particular type of cholinergic receptor known as a muscarinic variety that is found in the synapse (Wilson et al. 1995).

Significantly, nicotine prevents formation of the toxic beta-amyloid protein that causes neurofibrillary tangles and nerve cell death (Solomon et al. 1996).

Consult your physician prior to taking this product. Although the over-the-counter patches are weaker than full prescription strength, serious side effects such as addiction or habituation are possible. Would this really be a contraindication, however, considering the consequences of a progressing Alzheimer's dementia?

Because nicotine narrows small arteries, it is contraindicated in heart and coronary disease, mini-stroke syndrome, and peripheral vascular disease of the lower extremities. It is also contraindicated during pregnancy.

Nicotine is available by prescription in stronger-dose patches or as a nasal spray. Chewing gum, called Nicorettes, and lesser-strength patches are available without prescription. The patches are preferable to the chewing gum because of continuous, standardized twenty-four-hour release. Needless to say, smoking cigarettes is the worst way to obtain nicotine.

Tacrine (Cognex)—Prescription Only

Tacrine, initially marketed in 1993 as Cognex, is the first drug approved for the treatment of Alzheimer's. It works by inhibiting the anticholinesterase enzyme from blocking production of the neurotransmitter acetylcholine. This allows greater amounts of acetylcholine to be released within the synapses, which then prolongs the brain's ability to transmit nerve signals.

As continued neuronal death and hippocampal atrophy progress, the effectiveness of tacrine and all anticholinesterase-inhibiting drugs weakens (Riekkinen et al. 1995) because there are fewer cells to produce acetylcholine and transport messages. Accompanying this decrease in hippocampal brain tissue is steady decline in memory and mentation.

The greater the loss of brain cells, the less effective tacrine can be. A study in Norway reported that only 20 to 40 percent of those treated with tacrine exhibited benefits. Its side effects—inflammation of the liver and gastric distress—increase as dosage increases. It is recommended for mild to mildly severe cases of Alzheimer's (Arsland and Laake 1996). A study in England rates it 20 to 50 percent effective and notes its high rate of side effects (Eagger and Harvey 1995). A study at Johns Hopkins Alzheimer's Disease Research Center refers to tacrine as "effective" but cautions usage within clinical guidelines: slowly increasing dosage, serial monitoring of liver enzymes; and continued observation of side effects (Lyketsos et al. 1996).

The Alzheimer's Association states that this drug only helps a minority of patients. The cognitive improvements aren't significant enough to recommend it as a treatment for most Alzheimer's patients. Because of its side effects, "only a minority of patients with mild to moderate Alzheimer's disease can be treated with tacrine" (Kurz, Marquard, and Mosch 1995).

Donepezil (Marketed as Aricept)—Prescription Only

This is the second drug to be approved by the FDA for treatment of Alzheimer's disease. It was released to the market in 1996. Similar to tacrine, donepezil acts on the enzyme inhibitor acetylcholinesterase, which functions as a check and balance in the brain to prevent overproduction of acetylcholine. Aricept's blocking action on this inhibitory enzyme allows an increased amount of the neurotransmitter acetylcholine to be released into the synapse, thus increasing the brain's ability to transmit signals. Clinically, it is effective in mild to moderate disease but loses effectiveness as the disease progresses because there are fewer nerve cells to produce acetylcholine. It will not delay the progression of Alzheimer's dementia but will initially provide a degree of symptomatic relief.

One study showed that the symptomatic and clinical decline of Alzheimer's disease with Aricept was initially 50 percent less than in the control group (Rogers and Friedhoff 1996).

In another study of five hundred patients in Japan, 84 percent showed no increase in progression, and 50 percent showed actual clinical improvement. These results reflect a delay in reduction of symptoms attributed to the safeguarding of acetylcholine; however, they do not reflect a true delay in disease progression. In comparison to tacrine, donepezil is safer at therapeutic doses and without liver toxicity for patient's with mild to moderate disease, and it is less expensive (Barnerm and Gray 1998). Another study showed donepezil hydrochloride at a dose of 5 mg and 10 mg once daily to be effective for patients at the "moderately severe" stage (Rogers et al. 1998).

Still newer research shows that both tacrine and donepezil can exert properties protective of neurons, and, if so, this might possibly be of significance and contribute to greater clinical efficacy of cholinesterase inhibitors in general in the treatment of Alzheimer's disease (Svensson and Norberg 1998).

Selegiline (Prescription Only) and Vitamin E (Over-the-Counter)

Selegiline (also known as Eldepryl) is approved for the treatment of Parkinson's disease, and it was also found to be effective in the treatment and prevention of Alzheimer's. By blocking the transformation of toxins in the brain, it improved cognitive function, behavior, and learning (Tolbert and Fuller 1996). It also improved sexual function. It significantly prolongs survival and "is the drug of choice" in preventing Alzheimer's (Obenberger and Roth 1995).

As reported by the Alzheimer's Association, 173 patients with mild to moderately advanced disease showed significant improvement in memory after Selegiline treatment for six months, and progression slowed down even in those with moderately severe impairment.

Studies spanning two years with moderately advanced cases at Columbia University in conjunction with the Alzheimer's Disease Cooperative Study showed that over-the-counter vitamin E is equally as effective as Selegiline. Both are powerful antioxidants and show significant positive similar effects when used alone. When combined, they produced no greater effectiveness than either agent evaluated by itself. Compared with the placebo group, the participants took far longer to reach advanced stages of Alzheimer's when severe dementia, institutionalization, and death were evaluated (Sano et al. 1970). The ability of vitamin E to retard progression of Alzheimer's in moderately advanced stages represents a very significant and cost-effective step toward prevention.

MAOIs are enzymes in the brain that break down certain neurotransmitters such as epinephrine (adrenaline). Selegiline blocks the action of these enzymes and is in a class of drugs known as monoamine oxidase inhibitors.

A major side effect with this class of drugs can be a severe hypertensive crisis (high blood pressure) triggered by a reaction with sharp cheese, red wine, wild game, pork, and herring, all foodstuffs containing large amounts of the amino acid tyrosine. Tyrosine is an essential amino acid utilized by the body as a precursor for the manufacture of the neurotransmitters dopamine, norepinephrine, and epinephrine (adrenaline). Because tyrosine is so essential to the neurotransmitting system, it stands out as a very important supplement for their integrity. Deficiency is commonplace in Alzheimer's, and replacement of tyrosine is indicated since deficiencies cause nerve damage.

You may want to discuss the potential side effects with your physician if Selegiline is prescribed. Remember that vitamin E is equally effective and much safer.

Haldol (Prescription Only)

Haldol (haloperidol) is an antipsychotic drug that has been available for many years to treat psychiatric and nervous disorders, particularly schizophrenia. According to its pharmaceutical manufacturer, it is also quite effective in treating neuroses such as impulsivity, aggressiveness, mood lability, and excessive motor activity.

All of these neurotic (nervous) symptoms may be experienced through the intermediate and moderately advanced stages of Alzheimer's, and all are clinically responsive to Haldol. Of great importance, it has been observed that patients taking Haldol developed significantly less Alzheimer's dementia. Numerous research studies corroborate that Haldol inhibits the formation of toxic beta-amyloid plaquing (Higaki, Murphy, and Cordell. 1977).

This drug is an antipsychotic with side effects and is not recommended as a primary treatment for Alzheimer's. However, schizophrenics or other patients requiring long-term antipsychotic treatment, or those with neuroses as described above, should be considered candidates for continued Haldol therapy, particularly:

- if there is a genetic link to Alzheimer's
- if there is strong suspicion of early Alzheimer's disease
- if there are predisposing factors or markers
- if the individual is already diagnosed with Alzheimer's

An adverse effect of Haldol is its potential to inhibit the metabolism of the amino acid tyrosine (Braverman et al. 1997b). Tyrosine, you remember, is the precursor of the neurotransmitters dopamine, norepinephrine, and epinephrine (adrenaline). Since Haldol reduces tyrosine, by conventional reasoning it should decrease the neurotransmitters described above. Reduction in the amino acid tyrosine is shown to result in even more brain damage and thus enhance the progression of dementia. Yet this does not occur: Haldol continues to blunt the progression of Alzheimer's without any replacement of tyrosine. We thus have a paradoxical scenario: Haldol as both "good guy" and "bad guy." We conclude that it must be a very powerful agent to create, and at the same time, overcome deficiencies in tyrosine (which causes neurotransmitter damage) and still be able to delay the progression of Alzheimer's. Adding tyrosine to Haldol, therefore, should help to prevent neurotransmitter damage and synergistically enhance the delaying action by Haldol against the progression of Alzheimer's.

Prednisone (Prescription Only)

This time-honored steroid and potent anti-inflammatory was found to suppress certain imflammatory reactant substances known as antichymotrypsin and C-reactive protein. A small and tolerable dose of 20 mg daily was discovered to suppress the acute phase response in Alzheimer's disease. The "acute phase" is defined to occur when inflammatory cytokines (interleukin-6, also involved with stress) are provoked and amyloid plaques are deposited in the brain (Aisin 1996; Aisin et al. 1996).

Indocin (Prescription Only)

Indocin (indomethacin) is a potent anti-inflammatory drug that has been used for years to treat pain and arthritis. Research at the University of British Columbia revealed that Indocin actually arrests the progress of Alzheimer's (McGeer and McGeer 1996).

Thiamine (Vitamin B$_1$) (Over-the-Counter)

Experiments with thiamine derivatives on Alzheimer's patients (dosages of 100 mg per day) show some improvement in awareness, intellect, and emotion (Mimori, Katsuoka, and Nakamura 1996). Thiamine is essential for several chemical reactions in the brain, and autopsy shows the brains of Alzheimer's patients to be significantly lacking in thiamine (Mastrogiacoma et al. 1996). A study at the National Institute of Neurological Disorders determined that thiamine levels are lower in Alzheimer's patients than their counterparts (Gold et al. 1995). A lack of thiamine-containing enzymes disrupts certain chemical reactions in the brain and prevents one particular enzyme from utilizing glucose. Thus, cellular energy failure and cell death ensue (Heroux et al. 1996).

Melatonin (Over-the-Counter)

A burst of scientific interest and a corresponding increase in research about melatonin are showing so many vitally important benefits that they are included here:

Hydroxyl Radical Damage
The mitochondria within the nucleus of every brain cell that is affected in Alzheimer's shows evidence of a particular type of damage known as hydroxyl radical damage, and melatonin is a very strong scavenger that curtails such damage (Maurizi 1995).

Neurons and Blood Platelets:
Beta-Amyloid and Aluminum Damage
Besides scavenging free radicals and hydroxyl radicals, melatonin protects neurons from the toxic damage caused by beta-amyloid protein, which we know is the clumping of toxic protein between brain cells that attach to the RAGE receptors on the neurons causing neurofibrillary tangles and cell death. Evidence proves that beta-amyloid is also found to have harmful and damaging effects against blood platelets through a pathological chemical reaction known as lipid peroxidation. Moreover, aluminum has been discovered to be even more potent than beta-amyloid in causing lipid peroxidation damage of blood platelet membranes. Lipid peroxidation is an abnormal, unhealthy change seen in fat (lipid) breakdown by free radicals, and it plays a very significant

role in atherogenesis (hardening of the arteries), leading to heart attacks and strokes, as well as intensifying Alzheimer's.

A free radical is an unstable atom or molecule that has an extra electron (positive charge), or it can also be lacking an electron (negative charge). When a fat molecule in a cell membrane is attacked by a free radical, the fat molecule loses an electron and then itself becomes a free radical, but of a particular type known as a peroxyl radical. These free radicals perpetuate a process of creating new free radicals and continual damage.

When one atom of hydrogen and one atom of oxygen are combined with an extra electron, it creates a hydroxyl radical (hydrogen = *hydro*, and oxygen = *oxyl*), which is a rapidly acting and highly destructive type of radical. It is considered the most powerful of all radicals.

These processes of radical formations are never-ending, and they progress as chain reactions until they are stopped by radical-fighting scavengers such as vitamin E, vitamin C, or melatonin. Melatonin was found to be protective not only against lipid peroxidation of neurons and blood platelet membranes caused by toxic beta-amyloid but also protective against lipid peroxidation damage of platelets caused by aluminum.

To summarize, melatonin can effectively reduce the damage of lipid peroxidation caused by beta-amyloid and aluminum (Daniels et al. 1998). How great a role does aluminum really play in the pathogenesis of Alzheimer's disease? Even though many authorities and prestigious organizations discount its role, there appears to be sufficient scientific evidence to take another look.

Cholesterol and LDL

Melatonin decreases total cholesterol as well as the bad low-density cholesterol LDL (Chan and Tang 1995). Thus it offers protection against coronary artery disease, hardening of the arteries in the brain, stroke, and changes associated with Alzheimer's and vascular dementias.

Breast Cancer

A potential breakthrough in the complementary treatment of breast cancer is attributable to melatonin because it prevents cell membrane rigidity and inhibits lipid peroxidation (breakdown of supporting fat structures in cell walls). It has been found to be complementary to the anticancer drug Tamoxifen, and "these synergistic effects of Tamoxifen and melatonin in stabilizing biological membranes may be important in protecting membranes from free radical damage" (Garcia et al. 1998).

Melatonin also has an anti-estrogen effect that may depress the growth of breast tumors (Braverman et al. 1997b).

Cervical Cancer

Experiments with cancer of the cervix show a direct inhibitory action by melatonin (Chen et al. 1995).

Life Extended Thirty Years

Experiments on rats resulted in a life extension that would compare to thirty years for humans (Braverman et al. 1997b).

Melatonin is known to decrease with aging to the point where levels may be barely perceptible, and this may be a most significant contributory cause to the process of aging and the onset of age-related diseases, particularly Alzheimer's. This theory is supported by the fact that melatonin is the most potent hydroxyl radical scavenger thus far discovered (Reiter 1995a).

Cataracts

Cataracts are abnormal changes of the corneas that causes clouding an decreased vision. They are produced during the aging process by the depletion of the antioxidant glutathione that is normally present in the body. Melatonin has been shown experimentally to protect the eye and prevent the formation of these cloudy films over the corneas (Reiter 1995a; Reiter 1995b).

Macular Degeneration
Melatonin and vitamin E are both protective against free radical damage to the retina, the inside layer of the posterior chamber (the back wall) of the eyeball that sends impulses of vision to the brain through the optic nerve (Siu 1998). Cataracts are present to some degree of development in the majority of people over the age of sixty, and melatonin is effective not only in preventing them but also appears effective in helping to prevent macular (area of the retina that focuses images) degeneration, a leading cause of decreased vision second only to cataracts.

Oxidative Stress and Free Radical Damage
Studies of certain types of oxidative damage and lipid peroxidation damage to the hippocampus and other areas of the brain reveal that melatonin provides a protective role (Carneiro and Reiter 1998). Melatonin is more efficient in scavenging hydroxyl and peroxyl radicals than are other known antioxidants (Reiter 1995a; Reiter 1995b).

Oxidative stress is the result of free radical damage to molecules, and melatonin is able to reduce this resultant oxidative damage through several paths.

Ischemia-Reperfusion of Brain and Heart
An interruption of blood flow to the brain known as ischemia and responsible for TIAs (mini-strokes) causes pathological tissue changes that produce the clinical symptoms previously described

in chapter 4 under "vascular dementias." When the symptoms of a transient ischemic episode subside within minutes, hours, or even a day or two, it is indicative of blood returning to injured areas that had been lacking an adequate supply of blood, oxygen, and glucose. This return of blood is referred to as "reperfusion," and it is during these combined stages—ischemia (diminished blood supply) and reperfusion (restored blood supply)—that the harmful chemical nitric oxide is synthesized. The nitric oxide molecule is a very powerful and dangerous free radical. It spawns glutamate excitotoxicity in the brain that acts on the mitochondria to interrupt energy pathways and cause death of the involved cells. Melatonin prevents increases in neural nitric oxide, and by its action as a free radical scavenger it provides a protective effect on neurons throughout the ischemia-reperfusion process (Guerrero et al. 1997).

Toxins and Poisons
In pharmaceutical doses, melatonin is effective against damage from many toxic agents such as cyanide poisoning, paraquat toxicity, carbon tetrachloride poisoning, carcinogens, strenuous exercise, ischemia-reperfusion (return of blood to an organ after oxygen has been partly interrupted), and in reducing nerve damage in Alzheimer's (Reiter, Carneiro, and Oh 1997).

Melatonin Summary
Although functioning as a hormone, melatonin has been shown to wear several hats that deal directly and indirectly with Alzheimer's as well as perform vital roles in addition to those pertaining to Alzheimer's. Produced by the pineal body, a very small gland in the brain, melatonin is an amino acid derived from another amino acid called tryptophan. It performs as a neurotransmitter and

functions as a hormone. It inhibits toxic beta-amyloid damage to brain cells caused by lipid peroxidation, toxic beta-amyloid damage caused by lipid peroxidation to blood platelets, and lipid peroxidation damage to blood platelets caused by aluminum.

An extremely potent antioxidant, melatonin's scavenging properties against both the hydroxyl and peroxyl types of free radicals enable it to prevent cataract formation and protect the eye against retinal damage and macular degeneration.

Although effective in lowering total cholesterol and reducing LDL (the bad type of cholesterol), it is best known for controlling the circadian rhythms that govern our daytime alertness and nighttime sleeping patterns. Produced by the body after sundown, it peaks at approximately 2:00 A.M. and drops after sunrise. Evening dosing may be beneficial for sundowner's syndrome because it helps to overcome insomnia.

By bolstering the immune system, melatonin may also play a pivotal role in inhibiting certain types of cancers. It increases the effectiveness of the anticancer drug Tamoxifen in fighting breast cancer.

Usually taken in doses of 2 mg to 6 mg at bedtime, it possesses a wide safety range since amounts as high as 300 mg under controlled experimental conditions were shown to produce no harmful side effects.

Emerging with increasing importance in many areas and attaining even greater status as applied research continues to expose its potential, mounting evidence indicates that melatonin may be a life extender. In normal aging, its overall levels decrease but are significantly worse in Alzheimer's than in control groups.

The above merely touches on the current research and potential utility of melatonin. It would be prudent for all concerned to start taking this product in their fifties, if not sooner, to attain a fuller, longer, healthier life, and to help avoid cataracts, macular degeneration, and the four biggest killers. Its role is not yet fully appreciated as a supplement, and it may accompany Coenzyme Q10 and DHEA as the "miracle triumvirate" of the twenty-first century.

DHEA (Over-the-Counter)

DHEA, known as the "mother hormone," is produced by the adrenal gland and is the precursor of certain steroids and the sex hormones: estrogen, progesterone, and testosterone. Since DHEA is an important factor in keeping the immune system strong, a large drop in its level in the older population groups may help to explain, in part, why the incidence of cancer and several other immune-deficient diseases are greater in our senior citizens. Its levels are further decreased in many disease states such as Alzheimer's, breast cancer, and AIDS. Uncovered by research at the National Institutes of Health, the decrease in the level of DHEA in the Alzheimer's group is quite significant, with a loss 48 percent greater than control groups, thus compounding the fact that both groups already have considerably lower levels than younger individuals.

Increasing DHEA provides up to 48 percent overall reduction in mortality and produces a lower rate of heart disease in humans as determined in a twelve-year study at the University of California (1986). Administration of DHEA to rabbits with atherosclerotic blood vessels resulted in a 60 percent reduction in the size of plaque in the arteries as discovered in a study at Johns Hopkins University (Gordon et al. 1988).

DHEA is known to increase immunity by increasing the number of B cells that attack infection and the strength of natural killer cells in older male patients.

Although DHEA's sulfated derivative (DHEA-S) is protective of hippocampal neurons against glutamate toxicity, DHEA itself does not show this same protection. Moreover, levels of DHEA-S drop correspondingly along with DHEA in the aging process—and to even greater depths in Alzheimer's as previously noted. The action of DHEA-S is blocked by chemical actions, thus putting into question the role of DHEA in Alzheimer's disease (Mao and Barger 1998).

In both animal and human studies, lowered DHEA levels accompany the development of a number of disease states that evolve with aging. The negative effects of DHEA deficencies include:

- decreased immunity
- decreased life span
- increased incidence of several cancers
- loss of sleep
- decreased feelings of well-being
- osteoporosis
- atherosclerosis
- Alzheimer's

Immunity in aged mice was significantly improved by the replacement of DHEA, suggesting that this hormone plays a key role in aging and regulation of the immune system. Similarly, DHEA replacement stimulated osteoclasts (bone-forming cells) and lymphoid cells, thus retarding the progression of osteoporosis.

Another group of Alzheimer's patients were followed serially and given two specific tests every six months to measure multiple cognitive levels, the Alzheimer's Disease Assessment Scale (ADAS) and the Folstein Mini-Mental State Examination

(MMSE). They were tested comparatively at the same intervals for DHEA measurements. "There was a significant correlation between both the initial ADAS and MMSE [above] cognitive measures and initial DHEA level, with lower DHEA levels unexpectedly being associated with better performance on these measures." These results therefore cast doubt upon the use of DHEA with Alzheimer's patients to gain meaningful improvement in cognition (Miller et al. 1998).

The poor correlation of DHEA in Alzheimer's, however, does not detract from the multiple benefits noted above that can correct the deteriorating effects of aging.

Coenzyme Q10 (Over-the-Counter)

It is now universally accepted that disorders of energy production and electron transport in the mitochondria are a definite pathogenesis of Alzheimer's. We know that coenzyme Q10 activates the production and transport of energy in every cell in the body through its crucial role of aiding mitochondria to manufacture its energy in the form of ATP (adenosine triphosphate). Without this energy supply, the cell cannot function, and it withers and dies. CoQ, as it is called, is therefore the vital link in the production and transfer of energy in the brain and, as such, is protective against Alzheimer's.

CoQ is also a very powerful antioxidant that guards against free radical damage. It is normally found in very small amounts in every cell, but its greatest concentration is found mainly in the heart and then the liver, the two organs of the body responsible for heavy workloads. Concerning Alzheimer's, CoQ performs a double function by its role in energy production within the mitochondria and its protective role against mitochondrial damage by free radicals. The brain cannot function without CoQ. Its levels begin to decline past the age of forty.

The Brain

Coenzyme Q10 is particularly important in the brain for enhancement of cognition and memory:

- by correcting mitochondrial dysfunction
- by enhancing the metabolism of the mitochondria
- by enhancing the electron transport system
- by preventing toxic protein plaquing
- by performing as an antioxidant
- by its free radical scavenging
- by avoiding further neurofibrillary tangles and cellular death

Just as the descriptions of estrogen, melatonin, and DHEA unavoidably reflect essential benefits besides those associated with Alzheimer's, coenzyme Q10 commands the same attention because of the many advantages it provides to many vital areas unrelated to Alzheimer's.

The Heart

It is highly effective in the treatment of heart enlargement, angina, congestive heart failure, cardiac arrhythmias (irregular heart rhythm), myocardial ischemia (insufficient blood supply to the heart), and essential hypertension (high blood pressure). CoQ supplementation accomplishes all of these medically correctable problems by reversing an underlying CoQ deficiency normally found in heart disease, and by increasing the ATP energy supply produced by the mitochondria. It has saved countless numbers from morbidity, surgical interventions, transplants, and early deaths. Not yet well received in the United States, it has become the major treatment for heart disease in Japan, Europe, and other parts of the world, where it can be obtained by prescription only. In Japan alone it is the sixth most frequently written prescription and is taken daily by more than 12 million patients.

Life Extension

Claims of life extension are based on reversing the age-related decline of the immune system and hormone levels—DHEA, melatonin, estrogen, thymus, and CoQ. Supplemental replacement of CoQ will increase immune levels against heart disease, infection, and cancer by its antioxidant and free radical scavenging properties. Test studies done on experimental mice prevented the normal ravages of age and prolonged their life spans in human terms to approximately 150 years of age.

Cancer

Cancer is America's number-two killer. Many experiments worldwide are yielding significant levels of prevention and spectacular treatment results with CoQ, used alone or in combination with conventional chemotherapeutic agents.

In studies over the past two decades, CoQ has been shown to be effective:

- when used by itself with experimental animals in reducing the incidence, morbidity (suffering), and death in certain cancers and leukemias that were introduced
- in augmenting conventional cancer treatments and making them more effective

- in preventing or ameliorating (lessening) the horrible side effects of anticancer drugs
- in building up the immune system against developing cancer
- at high doses, and without any side effects, to reduce breast cancer with metastasis to the point where they "disappeared."

Obesity In a group of patients with a family history of obesity, there is a buildup of a particular type of fat known as "brown adipose tissue" (BAT) that contains numerous mitochondria and a great storehouse of energy. Burning up excess energy that is present in these huge brown fat stores is called "thermogenesis," and it can be augmented with CoQ. It is estimated that this group of "family obesity" patients produces only half as much "thermogenesis" as "normal" overweight patients (the overeaters), and that they have an approximate 50 percent CoQ deficiency. This group responds to weight reduction and obesity prevention by increasing their thermogenesis with CoQ replacement.

To summarize, ancillary to the beneficial activities it provides Alzheimer's patients, CoQ is proving to be one of the most vibrant, versatile, and complementary medications available for the control of heart disease, high blood pressure, certain types of cancer, immune restoration, obesity, and as a possible longevity agent. Caution must be exercised in both diagnosing and treating these diseases since there are many variables and potential pitfalls. Although CoQ is available for prevention and ancillary management, diagnosis and treatment are directed to professionals familiar with the disease states, their accepted conventional treatments, and knowledge of the extraordinary benefits of CoQ supplementation.

H₂ Receptor Antagonists: The Tagamet Class

H_2 receptor antagonists are a class of drugs that include Tagamet, Zantac, Pepcid, and Axid. They were developed to combat stomach ulcers and discovered to be very effective against the progression of Alzheimer's disease. These products were initially designed to prevent a type of histamine called H_2 from performing its normal duty of promoting the release of stomach acid. These blocking agents were employed in the treatment against stomach ulcers since acid was believed responsible for ulcer disease. Following blockage of the H_2, and their long-term use in the treatment of ulcer patients, it was discovered that the development of Alzheimer's and its progression were significantly delayed in the elderly patients evaluated.

As with long-term use of any medicine, however, it is appropriate to consult first with your physician.

WHAT SHOULD WE MAKE OF THIS?

The available agents just described above are all effective in the treatment of Alzheimer's, and several are very effective in other vital areas as well. Provided that Alzheimer's disease can be treated clinically, its progression can be not only retarded but also prevented.

Two medications, tacrine (Cognex) and donepezil (Aricept), provide symptomatic improvement, but they are unable to retard the disease process and they lose their early clinical improvement as dementia progresses. They are of help only until the advancing stages of dementia, at which time there is too great a neuronal loss for them to continue to be effective.

Of the other twelve agents, most are available over-the-counter and are inexpensive. In particular, the combination of estrogen, nicotine, coenzyme Q10, the anti-inflammatories, and vitamin E are incredibly effective in slowing down the disease process. If started early enough, they can prevent the clinical course of Alzheimer's dementia.

Aside from tacrine and donepezil, they are all effective in blunting the course of the disease. Using the equally effective over-the-counter agents as described in the "protocol of treatment" in chapter 12 can circumvent use of most of the prescription drugs. The treatment of Alzheimer's can be compared to a cancer: if it can be caught early enough, it can be arrested. The horizon is bright. We have progressed rapidly toward control of a previously mysterious and virtually hopeless disease. We have now reached a level of significant achievement and hope.

EXPERIMENTAL DRUGS

We will now consider a selection of experimental drugs from more than 3,000 new drugs in the pipeline. We cannot yet predict which ones will make the front pages and which will fall by the wayside. The FDA will approve only one in five drugs that make it to clinical testing; then it takes between twelve and fifteen years to get a new drug to the pharmacist's shelf. After years of research, three more years of preclinical testing are required, followed by three stages of clinical trials that last another six years. It then takes at least two to three years more before the FDA grants final approval.

According to the congressional Office of Technology Assessment, the average cost to get a drug from its inception in the laboratory to the pharmacist's shelf is $359 million.

Of the 3,000 drugs under current consideration, different classes of drugs and different modes of action are represented. Some of the following, applicable to Alzheimer's, have the makings of major breakthroughs of such magnitude as to be labeled "miracle drugs."

Anti-Spheron Agent NX-D2858

Spherons are "protein balls" detectable in everyone's brain at age one, and they slowly increase in size, enlarging 1,000 times by age seventy-five. Gaining such mass, they burst and become the amyloid plaques found in Alzheimer's and detected in the brain in the identical locations previously occupied by the precursor spherons. Investigatory research is in progress to develop an agent that can block this transformation of spherons into plaques such as the experimental product NX-D2858 (de la Monte et al. 1996).

Neotrofin™ (AIT-082)

An engineered drug similar in action to human growth hormone, it is now in its second and third stages of human clinical testing. Its uniqueness lies in the ability to mount a three-pronged attack:

1. It is able to prevent neurotransmitter brain damage caused by glutamate excitotoxicity.
2. It can mimic the action of astrocytes, brain cells that produce nerve growth factor (NGF) and two other protective proteins, including one called transforming growth factor.
3. It prevents degeneration of brain tissue and fosters

regrowth of neurons into damaged areas; results can be seen in as little as four days of treatment (Middlemiss et al. 1995).

Recovery of brain circuitry crucial to learning and memory, and also to function, is reestablished (Glasky et al. 1994).

Beta-amyloid Blockade

A chemically engineered protein has been created at the University of Wisconsin that binds to the toxic beta-amyloid and effectively inhibits this toxic protein from damaging nerve cells. Synthetic molecules have been engineered that are able to detoxify protein clumps. This approach represents a significant breakthrough in the prevention of a major cause of Alzheimer's (Keissling and Murphy 1997). This drug shows exceptional promise.

Kampo—SK, TJ 960

Kampo refers to Japanese herbal medicine. Research on an ancient prescription herbal mixture known as *saiko-keishi-to-ka-shakuyaku* (SK, TJ 960) unexpectedly revealed dramatic neuronal benefits. There was complete clinical disappearance of intractable nervous symptoms. It exhibited unheralded protective effects against neuron damage with regulatory action against adverse expression of genes and complete suppression of beta-amyloid-induced neuronal death. Channeled properly, this has the potential of being the true miracle drug of the new millennium (Sugaya et al. 1997).

Idebenone

Showing significantly superior performance in the Alzheimer's Disease Assessment Scale, this experimental product with a low side-effect profile promoted improvement in cognition and behavior. A synthetic analogue of coenzyme Q10, its efficiency as an antioxidant and free radical scavenger compares to vitamin E and is of even greater strength. Its capabilities range from scavenging several types of free radicals to inhibiting pathological peroxidation (Mordente et al. 1998).

Alcar

This is a chemical known as Acetyl-L-Carnitine that structurally resembles acetylcholine but is in a different class of drugs with a different action. It may slow the progression of Alzheimer's by its action of blocking the deterioration of cognitive areas of the hippocampus as seen in deficiency states. It also acts as an antidepressant. Its basic action is the transport of fat across the membranes of the mitochondria to supply quick and efficient energy (Braverman et al. 1997b).

Ampalax (CX516)

This drug, the first of a new class of chemicals, causes the nerve cells in the hippocampal brain segment to fire more rapidly, which results in improved memory. It preserves nerve growth factor

(NGF) function, preserves cholinergic receptors, and improves cell plasticity (Hampson et al. 1998; Deadwyler et al. 1996).

Propentofylline

Possibly a neuroprotective agent, it is reported to significantly increase cognitive skills and abilities of daily functions of both Alzheimer's and vascular dementias. It possesses beneficial activity against free radical and toxic glutamate damage.

Xanomeline

Xanomeline is in a class of drugs known as muscarinic receptor antagonists. Its action is similar to nicotine. It improves cognitive function, but surprisingly it has an even more dramatic effect on behavioral disturbances such as hallucinations, delusions, emotional outbursts, and agitation. Who knows? It may be marketed one day as a behavioral miracle rather than an Alzheimer's breakthrough! Scores of test subjects on four separate outstanding assessment tests all showed significant improvement in all the parameters tested including cognition, behavior (vocal, delusions, hallucinations), memory, and end-point analyses (Bodick et al. 1997).

Milameline (CI–979)

Currently in stage-three clinical trials, this drug also acts on the synapses to increase acetylcholine response.

Galanthamine

This is another acetylcholinesterase inhibitor. Like Aricept, it reduces the deterioration of cognition and shows some promise in the treatment of Alzheimer's (Fulton and Benfield 1996).

Metrifonate

Released initially as an agent against a parasitic infection, it was discovered to possess beneficial effects in Alzheimer's as a long-acting anticholinesterase inhibitor.

Exelon (ENA–713)

This is another anticholinesterase inhibitor designed for mild to moderately severe disease, and it is in stage-three trials. Studies of more than 3,300 patients are statistically significant and show impressive results. Its action is selective for the hippocampus.

CURRENT LABORATORY RESEARCH
OF THE HAIR-RAISING VARIETY

Strange paths are crossed on the experimental highways that often produce unimaginable vectors within the parameters of research. I do believe that some of these researchers would have made smashing debuts in *Star Wars* or *Babylon 5*. Their discoveries do them justice, however. They are to be commended on their wisdom and foresight in their quest for an Alzheimer's cure.

Testicle Implant into the Brain

Sound like science fiction? It's not. There is presently an attempt to transplant a special type of testicular "nurse cell" known as the Sertoli cell. The Sertoli cell is transplanted from the testicle of one species into the brain of another species where it is able to produce its own antirejection agent. Research is in progress in other centers using human embryo cells. Research at the University of South Florida is attempting to evaluate the eventual feasibility of cross-species transplantation into the human brain for treatment of neurodegenerative diseases. Theoretically, it can provide improvement, and this type of cell shows minimal rejection when transplanted.

Skin Implants into the Brain

In another experiment, skin implants modified with a gene to increase the amount of the neurotransmitter acetylcholine are placed into damaged brains of rats. The results are promising because rats demonstrated improved postoperative memory performance.

New Line of Mice

Known as transgenic mice, these experimental animals developed changes in the brain following implantation of the abnormal gene responsible for the amyloid precursor protein found in Alzheimer's. Using mice makes it much more cost effective to test new agents for Alzheimer's. After ten years of disappointing studies, initial success was achieved in 1995. Many generations of these mice now exist that will permit greater understanding of the pathogenesis of plaque deposition (Schenk et al. 1997).

Abnormal Skin Metabolism

The normally expected flow of cellular potassium and associated release of calcium from cells during metabolism of skin occurs abnormally in Alzheimer's patients, an irregularity that is not found in normal individuals or with other related dementias. The accuracy of this pathological finding is 100 percent in separating Alzheimer's from those with or without dementia (Hirashima et al. 1996). Hopefully, just gently scraping the skin will provide a very accurate diagnostic test in the near future.

CHAPTER 10

The Early Birds for Testing

Let's recap some of the information scattered throughout previous chapters about tests and markers, particularly the newer ones. If certain procedures described earlier are not included, it does not necessarily mean that those tests are no longer satisfactory. They continue to occupy a solid place in medicine as informative aids in differential diagnoses and they continue to be used. Only the most valuable procedures are covered here.

DIAGNOSTIC TESTS

A diagnostic test can provide a very high percentage of accuracy in identifying the disease based upon key elements of that test's sensitivity and specificity. However, not one test in medicine is 100 percent accurate, not even autopsy, although most people believe that it is. There are false positives and false negatives in every test and every aspect of medicine. The bottom line and final word is still your physician's. You depend upon your doctor's expertise to interpret all of the lab's test results, scans, and other studies within your clinical evaluation.

MARKERS

Markers, on the other hand, are indicators that show degrees of suspicion of disease. At times they can be excellent predictors of a disease state years before it presents clinically. But when either their sensitivities or specificities are not accurate enough to be diagnostic, they are instead considered markers.

THE IMPORTANCE OF EARLY TESTS

The ability to slow down the progression of disease is now within our grasp. The ability to prevent the disease is now attainable. The most critical step is early diagnosis.

The importance of an early diagnosis cannot be emphasized strongly enough. If the diagnosis is not made until advanced stages are reached, progression can still be slowed but not arrested. If the diagnosis can be made early enough, the disease can be stopped.

Tables 10.1 through 10.4 show the more rewarding tests and markers, tabulated to assist in propelling earlier symptoms into an earlier diagnosis.

Table 10.1 The More Important Diagnostic Tests

Test	Location	Accuracy	Discussion
3-D PET scan	University, hospital, or clinic	94% sensitivity 99% specificity	Has the potential of diagnosing Alzheimer's several years before onset. Extremely accurate. Considered diagnostic. Expensive. Some are private, but most are found in research centers of major institutions. Truly the "gold standard."
3-D MRI	Hospital or clinic	95% Accuracy	Measures size, shrinkage of the hippocampus and temporal lobes. Diagnostic for Alzheimer's. Differentiates it from other diseases and dementias. Best scanning modality after the PET scan.
AD 7 C	Hospital, clinic, or office	Approaches autopsy in accuracy	Test of cerebrospinal fluid (spinal tap) and urine. Best available procedure after 3-D PET scan.

Table 10.2 The More Important Markers: Professionally Administered

Test	Location	Accuracy	Discussion
Tau protein	Hospital or clinic	25% sensitivity	Early marker of disease. Levels elevate early in cerebrospinal fluid. Requires spinal tap. Considered good marker. Overlaps with other dementias.
APP	Clinic	25% sensitivity	Clumps out in the brain. Level in cerebrospinal fluid lowers. Needs spinal tap. Considered good marker.
Benton Visual Retention Test (BVRT)	Clinic	Very accurate	Predicts onset prior to cognitive symptoms. Excellent test. Superb early marker. Rates very high on testing scales.
Standard Alzheimer's Disease Assessment Scale (SADAS)	Clinic	Very accurate	Full test battery. Covers most disease parameters. Outstanding assessment. Top-notch battery.

Table 10.3 Home Test Markers

Test	Location	Accuracy	Discussion
Fingerprint patterns	Home	72% positive in Alzheimer's; 26% in controls	May predict Alzheimer's disease several years prior to onset of symptoms.
Sense of smell loss	Home	85%–100%	Can predict Alzheimer's disease two years prior to clinical symptoms.
Hearing loss	Home	Very accurate	Significant loss in Alzheimer's compared to counterparts. Early in occurrence.
Depression	Home	Very accurate	Occurs two years or more before cognitive symptoms. Significant if recognized early.

Table 10.4 Genetic Testing

Test	Location	Accuracy	Discussion
Apolipo-protein E4 (APOE 4)	Clinic	Poor	If one allele (copy) of APOE 4 is present, the chance of developing Alzheimer's is only 10%, even though the mutant gene is present in 30% of the population.
APOE 4	Clinic	Fair	If two alleles (copies) of APOE 4 are present, the chance of getting Alzheimer's increases to 50% by age seventy. Two mutant genes are present in 2% of the population.

CHAPTER 11

Treatment Essentials

Up to now, the treatment of Alzheimer's disease has been like putting together the parts of a picture puzzle. Enough of that picture is in place to reveal that treating, delaying the onsetof, and preventing Alzheimer's are possible. Old myths asserting that nothing can be done have been dispelled.

Since the original description of Alzheimer's by Dr. Alois Alzheimer in 1907, mainstream medicine has essentially looked on with morbid helplessness at this devastating illness. However, we are now witnessing the unfolding of a drama greater than Plato's classical story, "The Allegory of the Cave," in which the cave's inhabitants journeyed abruptly from a lifetime of total darkness into sudden bright sunlight.

As you have just read, massive worldwide research is on the threshold of discovering many newer agents for the improvement of Alzheimer's dementia. Although some are directed toward symptomatic relief, similar to Aricept and tacrine, others show spectacular promise of total cure.

ALTERNATIVE APPROACHES:
THE SWING OF THE PENDULUM

Research unmasks centuries old Ayurvedic and Chinese herbal medicines that are referred to in America as alternative or complementary medicines, although they are still treatment mainstays in most of the world. Several compare to, and in some areas even surpass, many modern drugs. They do this without the side effects common to Western medicine of anorexia, nausea, vomiting, rashes, diarrhea, vertigo, palpitations, bleeding ulcers, hair loss, and medication-induced death. Some of the herbal medicines are capable of readily replacing many of our current prescription drugs. Many others are well suited as complementary adjuncts to synthetic prescription drugs for the treatment of diseases such as arthritis, atherosclerosis, cancer, and Alzheimer's disease.

Modern medicines have been around for a relatively short time. The majority of these drugs have their origins in plants: bark, leaves, roots, and flowers. Modern medicine refines Mother Nature, synthesizes her ingredients, extrudes only one of many reliable components, and manufactures single extract synthetic drugs. In doing so, many of the natural checks and balances of Mother Nature are disrupted, left behind, or destroyed; this contributes to the many side effects associated with manufactured synthetic products. The natural ingredients of the vast majority of medicinal plants have negligible side effects.

Natural plant remedies and folklore medicines were the only pathways of oral and topical medicine in our nation's early days. At the turn of the century, there were four major branches of medicine: eclectic, homeopathic, allopathic, and osteopathic.

Eclectic (natural herbs) medicine was in the mainstream at the turn of the twentieth century, and it had several teaching institutions in operation in the early 1900s. Native Americans practiced eclectic medicine long before the arrival of the first European settlers, and effectively utilized multiple herbs and plant formulas. European settlers and Asian traders later introduced more. Many plant medicinals of the Americas were unknown in Europe, and their prominence persists today. As an example, echinacea, an herbal native to North America, is an important medication for the treatment of infections in Europe.

Homeopathic medicine was emerging at the end of the 1800s. Its theories and treatments originated in Europe, and it was particularly adept in the use of multiple ingredients. Homeopathic medical schools such as Hahnemann Medical College in Philadelphia were thriving. This arm of medicine fought fire with fire because it theorized that repeated subtherapeutic doses of an offending substance would cause the body to respond favorably. For instance, it employed minute extracts of animal organs directed to specific organ diseases in humans. And it worked. A similar therapeutic approach is seen with the modern treatment of allergy in which extracts of allergic materials—in the form of injections—are given repeatedly in infinitesimal doses to provoke the body's immune response and produce antibodies against the offending agent. Immunization to tetanus, whooping cough, diphtheria, polio, influenza, measles, and several other infectious diseases and epidemics follows the same homeopathic principles.

The eclectic and homeopathic branches of medicine were eventually engulfed by allopathic medicine during the first quarter of the 1900s. This marked the rapid change in the use of multiple but safe agents to treat disease by the theory of essentially using one single drug for one single disease. This same scenario was also taking hold in Europe and England. When modern methods of scientific investigation and research emerged, the majority of these time-honored, safe, and effective remedies were eventually expunged from the recommended pharmacopoeias (approved drug references) of mainstream conventional medicine. True, some remedy claims may not have been optimally effective, but overkill was in progress.

The *Pharmacopoeia* and the *National Drug Formulary*, the major drug references in the early part of the century, contained lists of all approved drugs including herbal and homeopathic medications. These publications were eventually superseded by the *Physicians Desk Reference*.

Although eclectic and homeopathic theories eventually fell out of favor, their practice did not totally disappear from Western medicine. Despite political maneuvering within the various branches of medicine, derision by rank-and-file practitioners, and the eventual near-complete dominance by allopathic medicine for nearly a century, centers of eclectic and homeopathic medicine held on and are again rebounding. Meanwhile, natural and herbal medicine—used effectively for thousands of years—continued to safely heal the ills of major populations in the rest of the world. Naturopathic medicine, an extension of eclectic medicine, gained popularity in America with emphasis not only on herbs but also vitamins, minerals, and natural body functions and treatments.

The first branch of medicine to evolve directly from the allopathic medicine mainstream was osteopathic medicine with its origins in heartland America just after the Civil War. Aside from surgery, it is essentially the first specialty branch to arise from allopathic medicine. Its founder, Dr. Andrew Still, was a Civil War surgeon. It originated at a time when barbers were still trying to compete with surgeons, a carryover from pre-Revolutionary days and early European influence. Hence, the red-and-white-striped emblems still persist in the front of barbershops today, a remnant of their calling cards in the early years of our nation. Osteopathic medicine was the first effort by conventional allopathic practitioners to recognize and appreciate the physical and structural aspects of medicine and the human body, and it was actually the beginning of holistic medicine. Its theories and practices saved the lives of many people during the worldwide flu epidemic of 1918, in large part due to use of an obscure technique known as the "thoracic pump," a procedure that propels greater numbers of phagocytes (white blood cells) into the bloodstream to attack infection and overcome pneumonia caused by bacteria and viruses. This is the branch that spawned chiropractic medicine.

After decades of political rejection by many members of the allopathic branch of medicine, the osteopathic branch has performed admirably and is again on a par with its allopathic sister. In some medical schools such as those in New Jersey and Michigan, students are permitted to take extra courses in osteopathic principles and techniques that cover aspects pertaining to the musculoskeletal structure of the body and obtain a D.O. rather than an M.D. degree In the early days of subspecialization in allopathic medicine, their osteopathic sister profession tenaciously held on to family practice, now referred to as "primary" care and "gatekeepers" in HMO medicine. Today we have too many specialists and too few family practitioners in many areas of the United States.

An old adage says, "With time, the pendulum swings." After nearly total medical exclusion in America, complementary and alternative medicines are resurfacing. We are witnessing the reemergence of the homeopathic and eclectic (herbalist) branches of medicine. In addition, the expanding naturopathic arm of medicine, with its emphasis on time-honored natural medicines and herbs and its similarities to allopathic medicine, is flourishing. However, we have not yet caught up to Europe where our over-the-counter "food supplements" (herbal medicines) are a major component of medical management and require written prescriptions. In areas of Western Europe, many physicians are prescribing alternative medicines in tandem with manufactured synthetic drugs, and in Eastern Europe alternative medical remedies are mainstays. America is definitely changing and coming around slowly. This does not deny, however, the efficacy of the majority of manufactured synthetic drugs; after all, most of the manufactured agents in current use originated from plant and herbal preparations. But when a natural medicine is as effective as a synthetic drug, has fewer side effects, and is considerably less expensive, it would be prudent to reevaluate your options regarding your freedom to choose the natural product.

As a board-certified practitioner with nearly four decades of clinical practice in family medicine and gerontology, I was aware, as were my colleagues, that many effective over-the-counter products were available. We were reluctant to recommend them. Alternative medicine was not taught in medical school when I was a student or throughout my tenure in medicine. Malpractice insurance did not properly cover items that weren't approved by the FDA, and the organized medical community frowned upon alternative and complementary medicine. In some states, medical boards censured physicians and even revoked their licenses for practicing alternative medicine. The FDA had its representatives march into offices, confiscate the alternative medications, and threaten doctors with prosecution. A physician practicing alternative medicine could not function without some degree of paranoia.

Many of us felt as if we were practicing in a medical police state, when time-honored and effective patent (over-the-counter) medicines that had been utilized for many years were recalled because they had not been "tested properly" by modern scientific standards. Fifty or one hundred years or more of clinical use and satisfactory results weren't sufficient. The FDA disregarded centuries of safe and effective utilization.

Some of these same items have been quietly reintroduced in the past few years. The medical theory of one drug for one disease adversely affected many time-honored and approved prescription medications with more than one ingredient, leading to their being withdrawn from the market by a well-meaning but arbitrary FDA. Ironically, it was permissible for a doctor to write the same medicines as separate prescriptions and allow patients to take them together. This didn't really make sense. It succeeded only in driving up costs for financially struggling patients.

Fortunately the pendulum is swinging back, and the public stands to benefit. What was considered blasphemy in medicine only a decade ago is now being taught in prestigious medical schools across the United States. Courses in alternative and complementary medicine are commonplace and being reintroduced with increasing frequency. A brilliant pioneer in this area is Dr. Andrew Weil at the University of Arizona, whose work with alternative medicine is impressive. Another courageous and outspoken pioneer is Dr. Julian Whitaker, the Californian who bravely challenged the system and successfully employed alternative methods for many years with his "Wellness Clinic." Dr. Jonathan Wright, whose knowledge of alternative medicine is unsurpassed, is one of the most outstanding proponents of complementary medicine.

The way in which politics spilled over into medicine is reminiscent of the McCarthy era in government. Fortunately, there are many heroes throughout the country who continued to practice their convictions in the face of such adversity. Basic and applied herbal research and teaching, as well as alternative approaches, are now being conducted at most medical schools and universities in the United States and worldwide. Other bona fide adjunct treatments are also gaining acceptance such as a relative newcomer in the field of osteopathic medicine known as "craniosacral" therapy. Endorsed by such pioneers as Dr. Viola Freymann and Dr. Jane Xenos in southern California, it provides spectacular results to infants and adults with musculoskeletal and genetic disorders and many chronic and intractable disease states.

The movement toward complementary medicine in America is so strong now that it is doubtful it can again be blunted. It's what the public and informed voters demand, and it is the trustworthy obligation of medical and political leaders to permit it. It will significantly reduce overall medical costs and improve the nation's health.

FOUR CORNERSTONES ENRICH
THE TREATMENT OF ALZHEIMER'S DISEASE

There are four cornerstones in the treatment of Alzheimer's disease that are predicated upon what we have so recently learned about it and what we are now capable of doing about it (see Figure 11.1). Avoidance of causative entities is very important and relatively easy to achieve. Intensive caregiving is vital. There are many available prescription and nonprescription medicines that we now know how to use to achieve maximum benefits.

Avoidance

Avoidance is an important preventative measure in Alzheimer's disease. We want to avert anything that will lead to free radical damage, oxidative stress, or electron transfer (energy flow) disruption,

Figure 11.1 Four Cornerstones of Treatment

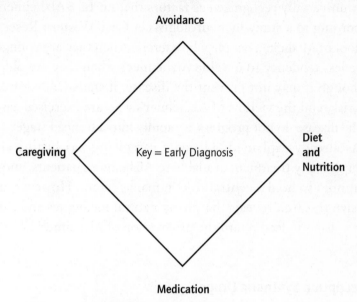

and new knowledge of several avoidable causes permits us to take judicious steps for better protection.

We know that certain items are suspected as causative agents such as heavy metals, electromagnetic waves, solvents, pesticides, and vitamin deficiencies (see chapter 6). All are avoidable entities. We know, too, that head trauma and high-fat diets, especially those high in saturated fats, are Alzheimer-friendly and can be avoided.

The lack of both mental stimulation and physical exercise are now universally recognized as factors that nurture Alzheimer's. According to a study by neurologists at Case Western Reserve School of Medicine, people who exercise when they are younger have less tendency to develop Alzheimer's when they are older. Although it may not prevent the disease, it statistically lowers the risk, and the victims of Alzheimer's who are exercised early in the disease do not progress as rapidly into advanced stages.

As already explained, adequate caregiving has historically been the only treatment available to Alzheimer's patients, and it continues to hold a central role in management. However, intensive research reveals that many natural medicines and synthetic drugs indeed retard the progression of Alzheimer's.

Prescription Synthetic Drugs

This subsection presents recommended doses and a brief review of prescription medications used to treat Alzheimer's. Included are the known beneficial items, but they may not be favorites in the treatment of Alzheimer's by some physicians who are unfamiliar with their effectiveness and may not feel totally justified in recommending them. They are presented here to broaden your knowledge of potential treatments and, hopefully, assist you in easing the burden of this terrible disease.

Tacrine (Marketed as Cognex)
Recommended for mild to moderate cases.
Dosage: 10 mg to 40 mg, four times daily.

Tacrine treats symptoms; it is not preventative of the disease. It is designed to protect the neurotransmitter acetylcholine.

Side effects: It can injure the liver, thus liver enzyme tests must be monitored intermittently during its use. It can slow the heart rate.

Donepezil (Marketed as Aricept)
Recommended for mild to moderate disease.
Dosage: 5 mg once daily.

The second drug to be approved by the FDA for treatment of Alzheimer's, donepezil, as does tacrine, protects acetylcholine and temporarily prolongs memory. Although safer than tacrine, neither prevents the progression of Alzheimer's.

Side effects: Abdominal distress, irritability, dizziness, itching, and hives.

Selegiline (Marketed as Eldepryl)
Recommended for all except very advanced stages.
Dosage: 5 mg twice daily.

Selegiline retards the progression of Alzheimer's by its powerful antioxidant activity. However, vitamin E supplementation is equally effective in inhibiting the progression of Alzheimer's with greater safety and less expense. It is effective even in moderately advanced stages.

Contraindications: Do not use with Demerol or other opiates, MAO inhibitors, or tricylic antidepressants.

Side effects: Use with MAO inhibitors, wine, sharp cheeses, or wild game may cause a sharp rise in blood pressure.

Haloperidol (Marketed as Haldol)
Recommended for early and intermediate stages of disease. For use in all stages if required for the treatment of psychoses.
Dosage: .5 mg to 5 mg, three times daily.

An effective drug in the treatment of neurotic and psychotic disorders such as schizophrenia, Haldol has been discovered to inhibit the formation of toxic beta-amyloid plaquing and thereby significantly retard the progression of Alzheimer's.

Side effects: There are potentially severe side effects such as involuntary body movements (tardive dyskinesia), Parkinson's-like tremors, hallucinations, dizziness, or seizures, but these are rare and usually manageable with proper dosing and close observation. They generally disappear when the drug is discontinued.

Estrogen

Recommended for all but late stages of disease.

Dosage: Premarin 0.625 mg daily, or its equivalent.

A female hormone, estrogen is an anti-inflammatory and antioxidant. It promotes the growth of nerve cells that produce acetylcholine, improves cognitive skills in Alzheimer's women, and retards the progression of Alzheimer's disease. It reduces the risk of Alzheimer's by 55 percent.

Prednisone

Recommended only at your physician's discretion.

Dosage: Recommended course is six weeks at 20 mg daily, then tapered down.

A very powerful anti-inflammatory, it can slow the progression of Alzheimer's in the acute phase response of the disease.

Side effects: With short-term use at such a low dosage, there should be no major side effects. It should not be prescribed if the patient has a history of tuberculosis or peptic ulcer disease.

Indomethacin (Marketed as Indocin)

Recommended in all except advanced stages.

Dosage: Maximum 25 mg, three to four times daily.

Indocin is a potent anti-inflammatory and is reported to actually arrest the progression of Alzheimer's.

Side effects: The most frequent are upset stomach with potential ulceration with long-term use. Possible liver toxicity requires intermittent blood testing. I have seen very few problems over the years with this drug and all have been minor.

Hydergine
Recommended for early and intermediate stages.
Dosage: 1 mg three times daily.

A mental stimulant, it does not retard progression or prevent disease. It may increase cognition in any age-related decline of mental capacity.

Nonprescription Synthetic Drugs

Anti-inflammatory Products
Motrin/Advil (Ibuprofen)
Recommended dosage 200 mg, three to four times daily.

They provide as much as 60 percent protection against Alzheimer's when started early in the course of the disease because they retard the progression to dementia. Orudis, Naprosyn, and Aleve are examples of other over-the-counter anti-inflammatory products available and suggested at over-the-counter strengths.

Side effects: Stomach distress, bleeding ulcers, and inflammation of the liver and kidneys are potential problems although much less frequent at lower, over-the-counter strength.

Nicotine

Recommended for early and intermediate stages.

Dosage: 7 mg patch. Apply once daily.

Nicotine slows the progression of Alzheimer's and improves learning by preventing toxic formation of beta-amyloid protein.

Side effects: Adverse effects can be observed by advanced narrowing of the arteries of the heart, brain, legs, or any other organ system such as the kidneys or bowel.

H_2 Receptor Antagonists

Recommended for all except late stages.

Dosage: At over-the-counter strengths, one each morning and evening.

Tagamet was the agent used in the major studies.

Pepcid, Zantac, and Axid are sister drugs of the same class that should show the same beneficial results.

Provides significant delay in the onset and progression of Alzheimer's.

Side effects: An interaction with a number of other drugs can slow down their liver clearance and elevate blood levels. It occurs mainly when taking the entire day's dose of Tagamet at one time, but since nonprescription strength is only 25 to 50 percent of full prescription strength, there is less chance for this type of side effect.

Diet and Nutrition

There was a time in medicine when it was believed that a person eating a healthy, well-rounded diet did not really require vitamin supplementation. We now know better. If we care about main-

taining an elevated immune system; avoiding heart disease, cancer, stroke, and Alzheimer's disease; remaining mentally alert;
and achieving healthy longevity, we should consider the latest
scientific research about large daily supplements of vitamins A,
C, E, selenium (ACES), and the B complexes.

We know that many nutrients perform in multiple ways. For
example, vitamin C, chromium, DHEA, melatonin, coenzyme
Q10, certain herbs, and the amino acid cysteine are all complementary to the treatment of Alzheimer's, perform multiple functions, and act as longevity agents. Add to these the herbs Ginkgo
biloba, Gotu kola, and ginseng, and you have the supplements
used for centuries throughout the rest of the world to attain a
long and healthy life. Modern research methods are confirming
many of these time-honored claims.

Adequate nutrition is essential to good health. Failure in this
area relates to malnourishment, hypovitaminosis, and a depleted
immune system. These deficiencies lead to further pathological
changes in the brain, which in turn accelerate the progression of
Alzheimer's.

Diet, geared toward protection from and treatment of Alzheimer's, has been a long-neglected cornerstone of this dementia. We now know that animal fat increases inflammation and
oxidative stress in brain tissues but that fish oils are protective
(Grant 1997). Substituting fish for meats and fowl is protective
not only against Alzheimer's but also against the ravages of cardiovascular disease. Seafood is high in omega-3 fats (alpha
linolenic acid), which, along with omega-6 fats (linoleic acid),
are essential to sustain life. Deficiencies support the development of heart disease, congestive heart failure, cancer, strokes,
vascular dementia, depression, and Alzheimer's disease.

Essential omega-3 fats are found highest in concentration in coldwater ocean fish such as halibut, herring, mackerel, and salmon and can be obtained commercially as cod liver oil and other marine lipid (fat) concentrates. Essential omega-6 fats are found in high amounts in sunflower oil and sunflower seeds. These are the "good fats" that keep down cholesterol levels, help prevent arterial blockage to the heart and brain, and help prevent Alzheimer's disease.

A deficiency of omega-3 polyunsaturated fatty acids is believed to be a cause of depression, and the lower the levels, the worse the depression (Edwards et al. 1998). Autopsy findings of brain tissues reveals decreased levels of polyunsaturated fats in cell membranes (coverings) of Alzheimer's patients compared to normal controls (Corrigan et al. 1998). Increasing the dietary intake of fatty acids provides significant improvement of these low levels in Alzheimer's patients (Corrigan 1991).

If an Alzheimer's patient is lacking in essential Omega-3 oils, supplementation by capsules would require an unpalatable number with every meal. An easier method is to use flaxseed oil, the only vegetable source of omega-3 fat that will match fish oil. The recommended dose is one tablespoon daily. For those who require more fiber in their diets, grinding ½ cup of flaxseeds daily (like grinding coffee beans) will supply the body's daily requirements of 20 g of fiber and sufficient omega-3 and omega-6 essential oils to meet all the body's demands. These items are readily available in health-food stores. Polysaturates, the "bad fats," should be avoided.

Ancient Greek stoic philosophy stated that anything in excess is harmful. This holds true for most things in life, especially fats. It is strongly recommended that total daily fat consumption does not exceed 10 percent of total calorie intake. Although this is less than the 20 percent recommended by the American Heart Association or the 30 to 40 percent average consumption of the typical (but poor) American diet, 10 percent is far more healthy, even to the extent of reversing atherosclerosis and unblocking narrowed arteries. Fortunately, packaged food labels now indicate the number of fat grams and calories derived from them, which makes food planning easier.

Research also indicates that lower caloric intake is an effective measure against the development of Alzheimer's as well as against heart attacks and stroke (Grant 1997).

Alzheimer's patients are known to have lowered levels of vitamin B_{12}, vitamin E, and other essential vitamins and minerals. Supplementation, particularly of the antioxidants C, E, and B vitamins (B_1, B_2, B_5, B_6, and B_{12}), is suggested over and above normal recommended amounts (see Table 11.1).

There are additional items that are lacking in Alzheimer's patients and require supplementation.

Phosphatidylcholine
Recommended for all stages except terminal.
Dosage: Liquid 1 tablespoon (3 gm) daily

This is the safest way to deliver choline to the brain to replace the lost neurotransmitter, acetylcholine. Lecithin and choline would be too highly toxic to ingest at such huge amounts. At 3 g dosing, it doubles the level of choline. It increases short-term memory at this dose, but is not as effective for Alzheimer's as anticipated.

Phosphatidylserine
Recommended for early stages.
Dosage: 100 mg three times daily.

It stimulates the availability of acetylcholine.

Table 11.1 Multiple Vitamin and Mineral Formula Geared Toward the Treatment
of Alzheimer's

Supplements	Suggested Normal Daily Amounts
Vitamin A Toxic effects heavier doses.	5,000–10,000 I.U. (International Units)
Beta Carotene* Converted later by the body into vitamin A without toxic effects.	15,000–25,000 I.U. Better if "mixed" beta-carotenoids.
Vitamin D_3 For bone metabolism but need some sunlight.	50–300 I.U.
Vitamin E*	400–1,000 I.U. For treatment of Alzheimer's, increase dose to 1,000 I.U. twice a day. Fifty-five percent effective in slowing the progression of Alzheimer's, even in advanced stages.
Vitamin C*	500–1,000 mg with each meal. Immune booster and antioxidant. Effective against heart attacks, cancer, strokes, and Alzheimer's, the four biggest killers. Surfacing as a longevity agent.
Vitamin B_1 (Thiamine)*	50–100 mg. Increase to 100 mg twice daily in early stages of Alzheimer's because it is deficient and supplementation aids memory and learning.
Vitamin B_2 (Riboflavin)	50 mg. Riboflavin is required for the metabolism of amino acids, the precursors of the fifty neurotrans- mitter systems in the brain. Deficiency is implicated in the formation of cataracts. Sufficient amounts are required for the proper therapeutic activity of pyridoxine (B_6).
Vitamin B_3 (Niacin)	40–100 mg
Vitamin B_5 (Pantothenic Acid)	50–100 mg. Plays a major role in the production of neurotransmitters, fat transport, and energy pro- duction inside every cell and maintenance of the immune system.

*These items may require supplemental dosing for treatment of Alzheimer's over and above the vit-
amin or mineral product you are using if the ingredients are substantially less than those recommended here. Dosage should not exceed the total daily recommended amounts. If needed to ease
compliance and improve nutrition, substituting liquid or powdered products is recommended.

Table 11.1 Multiple Vitamin and Mineral Formula Geared Toward the Treatment of Alzheimer's, *continued*

Supplements	Suggested Normal Daily Amounts
Vitamin B$_6$ (Pyridoxine)	50–100 mg. The most important of the B vitamins in the metabolism of amino acids and the fifty neurotransmitters; crucial in boosting the immune system and proper hormone levels. It is necessary for protein synthesis and the function of sixty enzyme systems (Hendler and Sheldon 1991). It is depressed by supplemental estrogen and requires replacement.
Vitamin B$_{12}$	100 mcg (micrograms). Deficiency is considered a major cause of mental deterioration (Hendler and Sheldon et al. 1991)
Folic Acid	400–800 mcg
Biotin	150–300 mcg
Choline	200 mg
Inositol	100 mg
Bioflavonoid Complex	100–1000 mg
PABA (Para-Aminobenzoic Acid)	25–50 mg
Calcium	500–1500 mg
Iodine	100–200 mcg
Magnesium*	500 mg
Manganese	10–25 mg
Potassium	100–300 mg
Zinc	25 mg
Copper	2 mg
Molybdenum	50–100 mcg
Selenium	100–200 mcg
Vanadium	25–100 mcg
Boron	1.5 mg
L-Cysteine*	500 mg
Betaine	100 mg

This compound has been described in numerous papers over the past several years, and it has been tested with several types of dementias and nonspecific "senility," providing some improvement in mental performance. When tested specifically in Alzheimer's-type dementia, it was found to be helpful only in the early stages, as seen in a study of fifty-one patients who were compared to a control group using a placebo (Crook et al. 1992).

Alternative (Complementary) Medicine

Ginkgo Biloba
Recommended for all stages except terminal.
Dosage: 160 mg daily in divided doses; anything less will not provide full effectiveness. Standardized to 24 percent of ginkgo-flavonglycosides.

Ginkgo biloba has been used worldwide for centuries. It is just now gaining acceptance in this country, offering several beneficial properties:

- It contains essential organic compounds known as flavonoids, terpenoids, and others that perform as scavengers against the free radicals believed to be a cause of Alzheimer's.
- Other studies show that it can delay the progression of Alzheimer's disease (*JAMA* 1997).
- It increases the acetylcholine neurotransmitter response.
- It increases circulation to the brain.
- It improves mental performance.
- It is known universally as the "smart drug."

- It is a potent antioxidant and destroys free radicals (Sastre et al. 1998).
- It increases oxygen and glucose supply to the mitochondria, augmenting energy production and nerve impulses.

It is available by prescription only in Germany, where 5 million prescriptions are written each year. It is reported as extremely effective in the prevention of early Alzheimer's disease (Heinerman 1996, 256). Total worldwide prescriptions are 10 million yearly, and this does not include most of the countries where it is available without a prescription.

Gotu Kola (Centella Asiatica)
Recommended for all stages except terminal.
Dosage: 60 mg daily of standard extract or 2 g daily of crude dried plant leaves.

Gotu kola has been used for centuries in India and China, specifically to improve memory and longevity (Mowrey 1986).

In treating Alzheimer's:

- It stimulates the central nervous system.
- It improves circulation.
- It improves poor appetite.
- It decreases depression.
- It alleviates varicose veins.
- It aids in sleep disorders, giving some relief to the sundowner's syndrome.
- It increases mental function.

It has been in use in France for over a century. In China it is accepted as a longevity medicine.

Ginseng

Recommended for all stages except terminal.

Dosage: 1,000 mg, two to three times daily.

Ginseng has been the most widely used medicine in China for the past five thousand years. It enjoys general acceptance throughout Asia and is gaining wider acceptance in Europe.

It has grown wild in North America for millions of years, and Native Americans recognized its medicinal properties long before the Europeans arrived. After being recognized by a visiting Jesuit missionary in the 1700s, it became a lucrative export to China. Daniel Boone made more profit in taking ginseng out of the forests then he did furs. It is said that John Jacob Astor amassed a fortune by exporting ginseng. Numerous ginseng brokerage houses still retain fur-trading names, although they haven't dealt with furs for many years. Ninety percent of all ginseng grown commercially in North America is exported to the Far East, and its use in the United States and Canada is rising dramatically.

It wears many hats:

- Ginseng is a mental tonic.
- It increases circulation to the brain, thereby increasing function.
- It improves reaction time.
- It enhances attention, alertness, and concentration.
- It enhances sex drive.
- It is an antioxidant.
- It is a free radical scavenger (Hobbs 1996).
- It protects against radiation damage.
- It shrinks cancerous tumors.
- It can prevent or abort a hangover.
- It acts as an immune booster, increasing white blood

cells and a chemical known as interferon, both of which fight infection.
- It lowers cholesterol.

St. John's Wort (Hypericum Perforatum)
Recommended for all stages except terminal.
Dosage: 250 mg to 300 mg, two to three times daily for depression and protection against infection.

St. John's wort possesses several beneficial properties:

Depression St. John's wort is widely used for the treatment of depression. As we have learned, depression is an integral component with 50 percent of Alzheimer's patients as well as half of all dementia patients. It acts by inhibiting the reuptake of the neurotransmitter serotonin at the synapse, and prolonging its utilization.

Anxiety Possesses mild tranquilizer activity comparable to Valium but without the side effects or habituation (Cass 1977).

Fights Infection St. John's wort has other beneficial attributes such as natural antiviral and antibacterial properties, both of which are complementary to Alzheimer's. Studies at New York University Medical Center and the Weizmann Institute in Israel revealed its dramatic antiretroviral activity. It is:

- *Anti-viral.* It fights the Epstein-Barr virus (infectious mononucleosis), influenza types A and B, and herpes simplex types 1 and 2 (Murray 1994).
- *Antibacterial.* It functions as a broad-spectrum antibiotic.

Immune System Stimulation St. John's wort, along with other immune-enhancing herbs, such as echinacea, astralgus, and goldenseal, all fight infection in a direct frontal attack against viruses and bacteria similar to synthetic drugs. In addition, their mechanism of action stimulates the immune system. While the synthetic antibiotics can only attack bacteria directly, they have no antiviral activity and no effect on the body's immune system. Unadulterated natural herbal anti-infectives are effective not only against bacteria but also against viral, fungal, and protozoan infections, something antibiotics are not. Some herbs also block bacteria by inhibiting a bacterial enzyme called hyaluronidase that breaks down a normal cell's resistance and allows the bacteria to gain entrance.

With overutilization of prescription antibiotics, bacterial mutations, and increasing resistance to these manufactured antibiotics, many herbal medicines are regaining some of their previous luster. In addition to far fewer side effects and proven efficacy against bacteria, viruses, and yeast, the natural anti-infective herbs offer something more than antibiotics do. They promote increased immune resistance by stimulating the release of white blood cells and interferon, which decrease inflammation and destroy these invading organisms. Although many of the prescription antibiotics are stronger than the herbal anti-infectives, many of the herbs are stronger than some of the antibiotics because of their broader spectrums covering multiple types of invading organisms and their modes of attack in boosting the body's own immune system.

In summary, there are many superb and lifesaving synthetic antibiotics, but bacteria are rapidly gaining resistance to these. On the other hand, the natural herbal anti-infective agents such as St. John's wort:

- fight bacteria directly
- Are also effective against viruses, protozoa, and yeast infections
- attack Epstein-Barr virus (mononucleosis, also called the "kissing disease"), influenza types A and B, and herpes types 1 and 2
- stimulate the immune system
- promote the release of white blood cells and a powerful substance known as interferon to attack infection and reduce inflammation
- block bacteria by inhibiting its enzyme activity
- show no bacterial resistance

Precautions when medicating with St. John's wort are avoidance of overexposure to the sun, use of MAOI (monoamine oxidase inhibitors) drugs, and other serotonin reuptake inhibitors.

Rosemary
Recommended for all stages where helpful.
Rosemary has been used as a brain stimulant for centuries since it has the ability to increase mental alertness, concentration, and memory. Although used as a spice in cooking and possessing antioxidant properties, it is utilized medicinally as an aroma, and modern research confirms its centuries-old claims. It may be purchased inexpensively in the aromatherapy section of most health-food stores, but many advocates simply grow a plant or two at home and rub a leaf between finger and thumb to express the aroma. Its use doesn't have to be restricted to Alzheimer's patients for stimulating mental alertness. Why don't you try it yourself? You may be more than pleased.

In fact, none of these mental stimulants need be restricted to

treatment of Alzheimer's. Ginkgo biloba, gotu kola, and ginseng—alone or in combination—are all in the realm of smart
drugs and stimulants for any walk of life; however, they are not
recommended for children.

Saiko-Keishi-To-Ka-Shakuyaku (SK, TJ-960)

This time-honored Japanese herbal mixture was recently subjected to intensive research and discovered—surprisingly—to
have several beneficial properties:

- exhibits preventive effects against stress
- is protective against neuron damage
- causes intractable nervous symptoms to disappear
- completely suppresses beta-amyloid protein–induced
  neuron death (Sugaya et al. 1997)

This startling capability of complete beta-amyloid suppression suggests we may be on the verge of a potentially major
breakthrough in preventing Alzheimer's.

For a complete comparison of both natural and synthetic anti-
Alzheimer's medicines, see Table 11.2.

Table 11.2 Anti-Alzheimer's Agents: Comparison of Actions

	Unique Action (See Previous Description)	Antioxidant	Anti-inflammatory	Free Radical Scavenger	Blocks Toxic Plaque Formation	Blocks Excitatory Toxicity	Promotes Nerve Growth	Protection Provided	Blocks H$_2$ Histamine Injury	Increases Cognitive Skills
Anti-inflammatory* (Tagamet, etc)	X	X			X	X		60%	X	X
Estrogen*	X	X	X				X	55%		X
Nicotine*	X				X			High		X
Tacrine (Cognex)										X
Donepezil (Aricept)										X
Selegiline (Eldepryl)		X	X	X				55% (Estimate)		X
Haldol	X	X	X		X	X		High		
Prednisone	X		X		X			High		
Thiamine* (Vitamin B$_1$)	X							High		X
Melatonin*	X	X	X	X	X			Very High		
Coenzyme Q10*	X	X	X	X	X	X		Very High		X
Tigan* Class of H$_2$ Receptor Antagonists	X	X			X			Very High	X	
Tyrosine*	X	X						High		X
Vitamin E*	X	X	X	X				55%		X
Ginseng	X	X	X					High		X
Gotu Kola	X							High		X
Ginkgo Biloba	X	X	X	X				High		X

*Crucial in treatment plan

CHAPTER 12

Treatment Protocols: The Essentials

It is obvious that no one person can take every single prescription medication, nonprescription medication, synthetic, natural herb, or vitamin and mineral that will offer some degree of help. Because of the severe nature of a dementia of the Alzheimer's type, everything humanly possible must be done to retard its progress and prevent its occurrence entirely. By necessity, this will require some mild megadosing of vital medications. However, megadosing medication is a chore even for the most robust person.

The most ideal treatment scenario would result from a very early diagnosis, a well-documented cause, and proven pathological brain changes. Then medical experts could zero in on and eradicate the basic underlying cause using fewer but more specific medications. How do we diagnose the pathogenesis? Is the dementia due to free radical damage or electron transfer disruption? Is there a long-forgotten head injury or unknown solvent exposure? Is the brain damage a result of a chronic inflammatory state or undetected vitamin deficiency? Are we combating an oxidative stress reaction or an unknown autoimmune disease? There is just no way to know for certain.

The following multifaceted protocol includes several medications directed against the causes and the pathological brain changes described in preceding chapters as specifically as our present knowledge permits. Unfortunately, there does come that unavoidable, painful, and guilt-laden time when that stage of disease is reached where nothing more can possibly help and the end is near—when it is fruitless to continue with any protocol. To be shrouded in denial or unable to accept the inevitable at the terminal stage of disease is unproductive. Rather, we must ask if the patient would want to continue in a pathetic, semivegetative state.

Nonetheless, doctors recognize that they are obligated to pursue every possible cause and prevent the metabolic and structural changes that destroy the vital synaptic connections and neurons. We are responsible for using every proven effective therapy at our disposal. If we can halt cellular destruction by shielding the brain from oxidative stress, free radical damage, and disruption of electron transfer, which are the end pathways of the multiple causes of Alzheimer's, we can prevent the disease.

CAREGIVING AND ITS TOLL

Caregiving today is the finest we have had to offer in the treatment of Alzheimer's, and it is key to any successful outcome. It involves almost constant attention to the following:

- good nutrition
- grooming
- cleanliness
- emotional support
- encouragement
- physical activity and a planned daily exercise program
- maintaining mental alertness

- avoidance of harm's way
- secured surroundings

As the patient's dementia progresses, the burdens placed on the caregiver to provide these things expand exponentially and can become overwhelming.

Physical activity is most important to the well-being of the patient. An excellent form of exercise is daily walking in the company of the caregiver. It improves the patient's bowel regulation, enhances muscle tone and strength, and helps boost the immune system. Exercise has been shown statistically to slow the progression of Alzheimer's. It is in the later stages of disease when the immune system weakens further, causing increased susceptibility to infections, strokes, and cancers, that inactivity and eventual incapacitation wreak havoc.

Aspiration of food and liquids into the lungs is commonplace due to increasing weakness, greater difficulties with feeding, more frequent recumbent positioning, and decreased ability to cough. These factors, along with a depressed immune system, are the major contributors to pneumonia. The caregiver must be alert to problems with food intake at all times.

Constant mental challenging can actually delay the progression of memory and cognitive losses. Numerous studies reaffirm that continued mental productivity definitely slows the progression of dementia. Encouragement of recent and past recall is helpful. Encouragement with writing, reading, knitting, and any other familiar activity is effective as long as the patient's orientation and mental responses permit. Repetition of activities and familiar surroundings are beneficial while change can be highly stressful.

Constant supervision is essential to prevent harm. Left alone, even with the caregiver in the home and giving constant supervision, the patient is still at risk. The major personal injuries comprise falls that cause bruises, lacerations, and fractures. Of those who fracture hips, 10 percent will die in the hospital, mainly from pneumonia.

Personal injuries to the patient aside, the entire household is vulnerable to the patient's mental lapses. Forgetting to turn off a faucet can flood the home. Turning on a toaster without inserting any bread or turning an electric stove to high and then walking away and forgetting are fire hazards. Only a lack of imagination can limit the list of endless possibilities that can and do occur. Caregiving is a twenty-four-hour-a-day job.

Caregivers eventually face physical and mental overtaxation. Their immune system also declines. Stress levels escalate dramatically, and frustration evolves with the daily struggles. More than half of all caregivers become depressed, and over two-thirds report anger and have a greater chance of developing heart disease from this pent-up anger, according to a study funded by the National Institutes of Health.

Anger is accompanied by deep and never-ending frustration because the greater one tries to assist, the less effective those efforts become. This can result in loss of the caregiver's self-esteem and an increased feeling of helplessness. The patient's progressive confusion, increasing refusal to cooperate, hostility, and eventual combativeness counterbalance the total effort expended by the caregiver. The well-meaning provider becomes anxious and tense, and may even suffer with insomnia, daily headaches, chronic fatigue, and a depressed immune system.

The duties of the caregiver eventually become so exhausting that either other family members are enlisted to relieve some of the burden or affordable outside assistance is secured. As the patient's dementia progresses and the caregiver's physical stresses and emotional dilemmas are stretched, often to their outer limits, caregiver guilt and depression escalate, culminating at the point when institutionalization is required.

NUTRITION

Everyone needs adequate nutrition. But it is even more important for patients who are debilitated; those suffering from infection, inflammation, or disease; or those who are immunocompromised with depressed immune systems from illnesses such as cancer or AIDS, or from strong medication such as cancer-fighting drugs. Alzheimer's is a disease state that itself is also beset by chronic inflammation in the brain and accompanied by toxic protein formation and excitotoxicity of neurotransmitter systems.

General

Intelligent meal planning is a cornerstone of treatment. Proper dietary needs must be provided. Three to five servings of vegetables and two to four servings of fruits are recommended daily. Supplemental vitamins and nutrients, although quite necessary, may not adequately fulfill all the body's needs. The body's requirements still demand the naturally grown antioxidants, vitamins, phytochemicals, and other nutrients besides commercially available supplements. The phytochemicals found in fruits and vegetables that are yellow, red, and orange are immune builders and cancer fighters. Leafy greens rich in nutrients are also immune builders. Greater dietary intake of fruits, vegetables, and grains will surely reduce the incidence of heart disease, cancer, stroke, and Alzheimer's.

Proteins

A minimum of 40 grams of protein daily are needed to prevent the breakdown of muscle mass with its ensuing pathological state known as negative nitrogen balance, or wasting. Protein requirements can be met with egg whites, skim milk products, fish, nuts, soy products, and other bean products and legumes. Reading food labels is an easy way to ensure that sufficient amounts of protein in the diet are supplied. Of these proteins, egg whites (or Egg Beaters®) and skim milk products are required daily since they contain all of the essential amino acids required for survival. Informative nutritional publications include lists of the protein content of vegetables, legumes, and grains.

Fats

Fat intake should be decreased because when metabolized, fats increase oxidation, the production of free radicals, and mitochondrial damage. As described previously, damaged mitochondria are interrupted from producing energy in the form of a chemical known as adenosine triphosphate (ATP), which consequently prevents electron transfer in neurons. This results in disruption of nerve impulses and cellular death.

A basic single molecule of fat has three binding sites. If no site is bound, it is considered polyunsaturated and referred to in medicine as cis fatty acids. If one site is bound, it is considered mono-saturated, such as olive oil. If all sites are bound, it is considered a saturated or polysaturated fat, and these are the bad fats that can play a contributory role in the development of Alzheimer's.

Saturated fats should be omitted. Fats with the least amounts of saturates, such as canola and sunflower seed oils, and other polyunsaturates, are recommended. Olive oil a monosaturate, is healthier for use in cooking because it has fewer tendencies than do polyunsaturates to hydrogenate when heated. Hydrogenated fats become partially or fully saturated and are therefore unhealthy. Hydrogenation means that a single hydrogen atom is added to the binding site of a fat molecule. This tends to harden a liquid (oil) at room temperature into a solid. This type of fat (hydrogenated) is referred to in medicine as trans fatty acids, and these are the really bad guys. Contrary to popular opinion, margarine (a trans fatty acid) is nearly as harmful as butter (a saturated fat). Some say it's even worse.

Some fats are healthy and necessary and are known as "essential fats" or "good fats," since we cannot survive without them. Two of these essential fats are known as omega-3 and omega-6 fatty acids. As the dietary intake of trans fatty acids increases, the body's level of omega-3 and omega-6 fats decreases (Hill, Johnson, and Holman 1979).

KEEP A SAFE DISTANCE

Avoidance is another cornerstone in the prevention of Alzheimer's disease. We currently have strong evidence pointing toward several potential agents that we know can cause or aggravate Alzheimer's. As deeply concerned as we are with the genetic inheritance factors that account for approximately 20 percent of the total cases of Alzheimer's dementia, we are equally concerned with the origin of the other 80 percent.

Several known and probable causes of the remaining 80 percent are avoidable (some were introduced in chapter 5; see Table 12.1 for a partial listing). Included in this list are medicines that have been used satisfactorily for many years such as Thorazine, Donnatal, and Bentyl. Although they are still very excellent medicines, their chronic, long-term use might be better avoided.

There are numerous environmental entities such as pesticides in our foods and drinking water, other chemical pollutants, and industrial wastes that in the future will play even greater roles in the pathogenesis of this dementia. To allow this to continue has the potential to be medical genocide. For example, a recent scientific report relates that the sperm count in men has been steadily declining at the rate of 1½ percent per year since the early 1930s. Although the reason for this decline is not yet clearly delineated, pollutants are suspected as a cause. Is there any question as to why more and more people are opting for organically grown foods and bottled drinking water? Looking back over the drastic changes in medicine and health over the past fifty years, I don't know that I could even come close to predicting the changes over the next fifty, other than to anticipate a cure for Alzheimer's and a further progression of longevity for both sexes.

I do not mean to engender fear in anyone, but I do suspect that a number of medications in current use eventually will be implicated as causative factors of Alzheimer's. On the other hand, there will be accompanying good news. Just as estrogen, vitamin E, the anti-inflammatories, nicotine, and other agents have been found to significantly slow the progression of Alzheimer's and thus pre-

Table 12.1 Avoidable Potential Causes of Alzheimer's

Potential Causes	Risk Factors
Stress	Prolonged and chronic
Head injury	Greater risk with unconsciousness and possession of APOE 4
Thorazine	Chronic use of some antihistamines, such as chlorpromazine (Thorazine)
Electromagnetic fields	Emerging as a cause of Alzheimer's
Solvent exposure	Agents such as toluene, benzene, and ketones
Zinc exposure	New evidence links zinc to Alzheimer's
Donnatal and Bentyl	Prolonged or chronic use of the anticholinergic class of medicine
Aluminum	Is the aluminum door totally closed?

vent it, other items in current use will eventually emerge with equal and hopefully stronger properties.

THE MORE IMPORTANT MEDICATIONS

Tables 12.2 through 12.5 present the more important medications for the treatment and prevention of Alzheimer's.

A strong, therapeutic multivitamin and mineral combination is required to ensure peak performance of all other medications utilized in treatment as well as all of the body's metabolic functions. The role of the B vitamins are essential in the metabolism of amino acids and the production of neurotransmitters.

Estrogen, as we have learned, is an absolutely crucial supplement for every postmenopausal woman unless contraindicated.

Vitamin E, nicotine, the anti-inflammatories (such as ibuprofen), and the Tagamet class of medicines have a proven track record because of their actions against the known avenues of pathogenesis in the brain. Unless there are contraindications to any of these agents, all four are required daily since they can really be lifesaving.

Coenzyme Q10, a substance able to enter the nucleus of every cell in the body, protects the mitochondria from damage, disruption of energy transfer, and cell death.

Autopsy reveals that tyrosine, an essential amino acid, is lacking in Alzheimer's patients. It is the precursor of adrenaline and other neurotransmitters. Vital chemical reactions malfunction in the mitochondria by the tyrosine-dependent neurotransmitters when a deficiency is present. Cellular brain death occurs, and this further intensifies the Alzheimer process.

Vitamin B_1 deficiencies in Alzheimer's patients are recognized at autopsy. Since it is a vital ingredient for several enzyme reactions in the brain, replacement will retard the progression of the disease.

Melatonin is another amino acid that is necessary for several biological reactions. As described previously, it is an antioxidant, neurotransmitter, and hydroxyl radical scavenger. It functions as a hormone, is referred to as a life extender, and has several other beneficial functions. It is best known for its ability to regulate the body's day-night clock. This will allow both the patient and the family to sleep at night.

Ginkgo biloba, gotu kola, and ginseng are time-honored herbal medicines for Alzheimer's, and they continue to remain the mainstay of treatment throughout most of the world. Although they have not been listed below as crucial, their addition to the treatment regimen is synergistic and effective.

Table 12.6 ("bare bones" agents) includes the ten most crucial and effective agents in our current arsenal that are capable of preventing Alzheimer's.

The essential treatment items are of nearly equal importance. The B vitamins are essential for the "bare bones" agents to function at full capacity. Frankly, they are so important that they should also be described as crucial.

The herbs that are described as very strongly recommended have been remedies for centuries, and they still remain the choice of treatment for Alzheimer's disease throughout the world. Their efficacy cannot be minimized.

By this time you should be able to treat Alzheimer's as if you yourself were a professional. I am sure that you have a firm grasp of the symptoms outlined in chapter 3 and the causes presented in chapter 6. You have an understanding of the Alzheimer's-related dementias in chapter 4. You are familiar with the many genetic causes presented in chapter 7. You are well aware of the little-known but very important markers for the disease found in chapter 8, and of the significant tests described in chapter 10.

The research unveiled in chapter 9, the essentials of treatment proposed in chapter 11, and the present protocols of treatment designed in this chapter are keys to the prevention of Alzheimer's. In view of the huge amount of medical material presented, you may benefit by reviewing the core chapters, 9, 11, and 12 from time to time.

As revealed throughout this book, a multifaceted (diverse) treatment approach is currently required in order to provide the greatest possible protection against the known causes and pathogenic changes leading to Alzheimer's disease. This treatment plan is designed to prevent these pathways of cellular destruction. Intensive research points to several potentially spectacular

Table 12.2 Summary of Proven Effective Prescription Medications*

Prescription	Status	Discussion
Aricept (Donepezil) 10 mg to 40 mg four times daily	Very effective	For symptomatic control. Improves cognition but loses its effect in advanced stages and does not retard progression. Can cause liver toxicity.
Estrogen (Premarin) 0.625 mg daily or its equivalent	Crucial 55% effective	A must for all women past menopause unless contraindicated. Antioxidant. Anti-inflammatory. Cardioprotective. Many life-prolonging properties.
Prednisone 20 mg once daily for short duration	Very effective	Very powerful anti-inflammatory. Will arrest progression. Side effects with heavy and prolonged use. Must be taken under physician supervision.
Indocin (Indomethacin) 25 mg four times daily	Very effective	Reportedly able to arrest progression of disease. Mild side effects. Possibly the anti-inflammatory of choice if closely watched by physician.
Hydergine 1 mg three times daily	Somewhat effective	Symptomatic. Improves cognition in most dementias. Not terribly popular.
Haldol (Haloperidol) 0.5 mg to 5 mg three times daily	Very effective against Alzheimer's	Powerful psychotropic drug for schizophrenia and other mental disorders. Remarkably effective in retarding progression of Alzheimer's. Drug of choice in Alzheimer's if medication is required for treatment of psychoses or neuroses. Blocks the formation of beta-amyloid plaquing.
Selegiline (Eldepryl) 5 mg daily	Very effective	Parkinson's disease medication. Able to retard progression and offer prevention of Alzheimer's. Strong antioxidant. In class of MAOI drugs. Side effects with Haldol and tyrosine-containing foods. Vitamin E is much safer and equally effective in treating Alzheimer's.

*All medications in Table 12.2 are by prescription only. Discuss proven benefits against possible side effects with your physician.

Table 12.3 Summary of Proven Effective Nonprescription Medications*

Medication	Status	Discussion
Ibuprofen 200 mg daily	Crucial 60% Effective	A must unless contraindicated by allergy or GI bleed. Check with physician if in doubt. Anti-inflammatory. Blocks excitotoxicity and H_2 histamine effects. Helps prevent Alzheimer's disease.
Tagamet, Axid Pepcid, Zantac morning and evening	Crucial	Over-the-counter strength recommended. It protects against toxic protein formation. Helps prevent Alzheimer's disease.
Nicotine patch 7 mg or 14 mg once daily	Crucial	A must unless contraindicated by vascular disease or allergy. Check with physician. It protects against toxic protein formation. Helps prevent Alzheimer's disease.
Coenzyme Q10 30 mg to 60 mg daily	Crucial	Enhances brain cell function. Improves cognition. Enters mitochondria of every cell in the body. Aids electron (energy) transfer. Prevents plaquing and excitatory cell death, seen in Alzheimer's.
Tyrosine 1 g to 2 g daily	Crucial	Essential for neurotransmitters. Avoid MAO inhibitor-type medications (Selegiline). Lacking in Alzheimer's. Must supplement.
Melatonin 3 mg one hour before bedtime	Crucial	Helps circadian rhythms. Allows family to sleep. Antioxidant. Neurotransmitter. Hydroxyl radical scavenger. Immune booster. Blocks beta-amyloid plaquing.

*Avoid any of these medicines if there is a history of contraindication or side effects. Recommended doses are only guidelines. Fewer side effects occur at these levels than at full prescription strengths of the anti-inflammatory and Tagamet families and nicotine. Coenzyme Q10 is safe past 300 mg daily. Tyrosine is safe at 5 g daily. Melatonin has been dosed at 200 mg per night experimentally. If there are any questions, check with your physician. Dosage may need to be adjusted up or down depending upon individual case history and the stage of disease. Adjustment is simple but should be under physician advisement.

Table 12.4 Summary of Vitamin Supplement Requirements: Exceeding "Normal"*

Medication	Status	Discussion
Vitamin C 1,000 mg three times daily	Essential	Strong antioxidant, free radical scavenger, immune builder. Anticancer properties. Proven life extender.
Vitamin E 1,000 mg twice daily	Crucial 55% Effective	Of greatest importance. 55% effective against Alzheimer's. Can even retard advanced cases. Anti-inflammatory, etc.
Multivitamin/Mineral Therapeutic strength daily	Crucial	Essential for all chemical reactions. For peak performance of all medications and all metabolic functions in the body. Requires proper strength.
Vitamin B₁ (Thiamine) 100 mg twice daily	Crucial	Essential for major chemical and enzyme reactions in the brain. Autopsy reveals deficient levels.
Vitamin B₂ (Riboflavin) 50 mg daily	Essential	Required for the production of neurotransmitters.
Vitamin B₅ (Pantothenic Acid) 50 to 100 mg daily	Essential	Plays a major role in the production of neurotransmitters.
Vitamin B₆ (Pyridoxine) 50 mg to 100 mg daily	Essential	Required for over sixty enzyme functions in the body.
Vitamin B₁₂ 1,000 mcg monthly by injection or sublingual	Essential	Normally low in Alzheimer's. Prevents pernicious anemia and dementia. Maintains nerve sheath. Can omit if blood levels are mid-range to high.
Flaxseed oil One tablespoon daily	Essential	Contains therapeutic amounts of omega-3, omega-6, and other essential fatty acids. Prevents arterial blockage in the heart and brain, and slows Alzheimer's. Helps prevent depression.

*When selecting your therapeutic multivitamin, read the label carefully to ensure that recommended amounts (mg, g) are present. You may have to shop around to find a satisfactory multivitamin. If your purchase contains amounts lower than that recommended for any item, you may have to add another supplement. For example, if your multivitamin has only 50 mg of vitamin B₁, you will want to supplement it with an additional 150 mg daily. Be careful not to accidentally overdose a nutrient if doubling up one or more similar items.

Table 12.5 Summary of Time-Honored and Worldwide Effective Herbs

Medication	Status	Discussion
Ginkgo Biloba 80 mg twice daily	Very strongly recommended	The "smart drug." Worldwide use. Retards progression of Alzheimer's. Prescribed as a life extender throughout the rest of the world.
Gotu Kola extract 60 mg twice daily Or dried leaves 1 g twice daily	Very strongly recommended	Worldwide use. Circulatory stimulant. Improves cognition.
Ginseng 1 g twice daily	Very strongly recommended	Centuries of indisputable help. Many benefits. Worldwide use.
St. John's wort 250 mg daily	Strongly recommended where indicated	Very strong antidepressant. Reported to be as effective as Prozac without the side effects. Also antiviral and antibacterial.
Rosemary Aromatherapy	Effective	Increases mental alertness, cognition.

breakthroughs, and we already have several approaches that help us prevent the progression of Alzheimer's.

Although the suggestions regarding mild megadosing may raise an eyebrow or two, we are actually utilizing the only known, proven, and currently effective treatment strategies in the battle against Alzheimer's. We eagerly anticipate the day when a one- or two-drug regimen will prevent Alzheimer's disease. Experimentally, there are many agents that show promise. Of the medicines in development and undergoing clinical trials, two types show particularly great potential. One inhibits toxic protein from damaging the neuron and preventing cell death by employing engineered synthetic molecules that detoxify the beta-amyloid protein clumps. The other, Neotrofin™ (AIT-082), acting mainly on the hippocampus and preventing glutamine toxicity, preserves the

Table 12.6 The "Bare Bones": The Crucial Ten*

Medication	Status	Discussion
Estrogen (Premarin) 0.625 mg daily or its equivalent	Crucial 55% effective against Alzheimer's	A must for all women past menopause unless contraindicated. Antioxidant. Anti-inflammatory. Aids acetylcholine. Slows progression of Alzheimer's in advanced stages. Retards osteoporosis, heart attack. Alzheimer's preventative.
Ibuprofen 200 mg three to four times daily	Crucial 60% effective against Alzheimer's	Unless contraindicated by GI bleed or allergy. Check with physician. Slows progression. Ibuprofen used in major studies. Other anti-inflammatories available. A must. Helps prevent Alzheimer's disease.
Tagamet, Axid, Pepcid, or *Zantac* Over-the-counter strength. morning and evening	Crucial	Retards progression. A must. Prevents toxic protein. Helps prevent Alzheimer's disease.
Nicotine Patch 7 mg or 14 mg patch daily	Crucial	Unless contraindicated by vascular disease or allergy—check with physician. Retards progression. Helps prevent Alzheimer's disease.
Coenzyme Q10 30–60 mg daily	Crucial	Enhances brain cell function. Improves cognition. Enhances energy and electron transfer. Protects mitochondria from injury and death. Anti-excitotoxic.
Tyrosine 1–2 g daily	Crucial	Essential for neurotransmitters. Deficient in Alzheimer's. Avoid MAO inhibitor-type medications.
Vitamin E 1,000 mg twice daily	Crucial 55% effective against Alzheimer's	Of greatest importance. Can help prevent Alzheimer's disease if started early. Can even retard advanced cases. Antioxidant. Anti-inflammatory. A must!

Table 12.6 The "Bare Bones": The Crucial Ten, *continued*

Medication	Status	Discussion
Multivitamin/Mineral Therapeutic strength daily	Crucial	Essential for all chemical reactions in the entire body and for effectiveness of all medications taken.
Vitamin B₁ (Thiamine) 100 mg twice daily	Crucial	Essential for major chemical reactions in the brain. Revealed by autopsy to be deficient in Alzheimer's.
Melatonin 3–6 mg one hour before bedtime	Crucial	Free radical scavenger, antioxidant, beta-amyloid blocker, immune booster, life extender. Controls circadian rhythms.

*Observe all previous recommendations regarding possible side effects, allergy, dosage limitations, and physician advisement. Read manufacturers' recommendations and precautions on all medications. Of these ten *crucial* items, only estrogen is by prescription and not recommended for men. The other nine items are over-the-counter and readily accessible for an easy and uncomplicated course of treatment at home.

loss of nerve growth hormone and fosters regrowth of brain cells into damaged areas. It not only prevents, but also reverses and restores memory deficits. Its future potential goes beyond Alzheimer's and, indeed, holds promise of helping patients with age-related memory deficits, too.

There is nothing else we know of or can do at present to further retard the progression or completely prevent the disease. Whatever effort it takes to follow the treatment plan as outlined in this book is worth it, as it improves the quality of life of all involved in an Alzheimer's patient's challenges. The effectiveness of these agents in this regimen is stunning: up to 60 percent for ibuprofen, 55 percent for vitamin E, and 55 percent for estrogen. Combined, they are synergistic: they complement one another and provide greater protection.

All are further enhanced by the action of other agents listed in the core chapters. Even though many of the patients who were tested with these "critical" medicines (vitamin E, estrogen, anti-inflammatories, Tagamet, nicotine) were already in advanced stages when the medications were started, these agents still showed evidence of slowing down the progress of the disease. If the burden of multiple daily medications appears too great an encumbrance, ask yourself if the patient's quality of life is worth it, and if the family's physical endurance and mental health are worth the effort. I know that they are. Clearly, if the disease is diagnosed early enough and the treatment started in time, its progression can be delayed sufficiently for the person to lead a normal, healthy, full life. We can outlive the disease. We can prevent it.

Thank you for listening and trying.

I wish you well, and many years of a happy, healthy, productive, and satisfying life.

Glossary

Acetylcholine A chemical of the cholinergic neurotransmitting system. It is responsible for the transfer of nerve impulses across the synapses.

AD 7 C This is the most significant cerebrospinal fluid test to date, closely matching that of autopsy for accuracy. It is the measurement of a specific brain protein that shows a ten-fold increase in the Alzheimer's. Can also be evaluated utilizing a urine test.

Allele Genes normally occur in pairs—one inherited from each parent—and they are carried in the same location on each paired chromosome of every cell. If a genetic mutation creates an extra copy of itself, this copy is called an allele.

Aluminum Held the spotlight for many years as a primary cause of Alzheimer's disease. Although officially discounted now as a cause, it still remains controversial.

Alzheimer's Disease A chronic, progressive deterioration of the brain leading to dementia, incapacitation, and death. Responsible for 70 percent of all dementia-related deaths.

Alzheimer's-Related Dementias A group of dementias of various etiologies (causes) that overlap or mimic the symptoms of Alzheimer's dementia. They can be very difficult to differentiate or separate clinically from one another.

Amyloid Precursor Protein (APP) A protein that clumps in the brain, causing its levels to decrease in the cerebrospinal fluid. This makes it a marker for predicting the presence of Alzheimer's disease. The genetic mutation is located on chromosome #21.

Anticholinesterase A "check and balance" enzyme responsible for regulating and lowering levels of acetylcholine and preventing overproduction.

Antichymotrypsin An inflammatory reactant chemical in the body.

Antihistamines Chemicals, synthetics, and natural herbs, that possess anti-allergic properties. They reduce the proliferation of histamine H_1—responsible for allergic symptoms.

Antioxidant Chemicals found in fruits, vegetables, and herbs, that prevent damage from free radicals and chemical oxidation. These destructive processes involve Alzheimer's, cardiovascular, and other disease states.

Anxiolytics Synthetic chemicals and herbs that reduce anxiety.

APOE 4 The subtype #4 of apolipoprotein E. Its copy is a genetic precursor of Alzheimer's. Although 30 percent of the population carry this allele, only 10 percent of carriers will develop the disease; 90 percent will not.

Apolipoprotein E A molecule that carries four different genetic subtypes, referred to as E1, E2, E3, E4.

Atrophy Shrinkage of tissues. It is seen particularly in the hippocampus in Alzheimer's (the brain segment involved with learning and memory) and also in the temporal lobes of the brain.

Autoimmune Disease An inflammatory state of the body in which the body's own antibodies attack it and cause irreparable damage and destruction to certain predetermined, selected tissues.

Autopsy Study of the body and its tissues and fluids after death.

Autotoxic Process A chronic inflammation of organ systems that can contribute to cellular death in the brain.

BEAM Brain Electrical Activity Mapping test. Evaluates the velocity of brain waves.

BVRT Benton Visual Retention Test. Capable of predicting Alzheimer's prior to the onset of cognitive symptoms which makes it a good marker of disease.

Caregivers Those who render day-to-day care and management of Alzheimer's patients. They are usually close family members.

CAT Scan A computerized axial tomography type of x-ray scan that is more accurate concerning the study of bone. When employed for the study of the brain, it is more diagnostic for circulatory disease than for Alzheimer's.

Cerebral Hemispheres Two major bilateral segments of the brain that manifest some involvement with Alzheimer's.

Cerebrospinal Fluid A fluid that bathes the brain, spinal cord, and canal. It is important in Alzheimer's for the measurement of disease-related proteins found in this fluid.

Cholinergic Relates to the parasympathetic nervous system which utilizes acetylcholine as a neurotransmitter.

Cholinergic Nerve Receptor Type of nerve receptor of the parasympathetic nervous system. Located at the synapse, it involves the release and reuptake of the neurotransmitter acetylcholine.

Chromosome #1 The mutated gene found on chromosome #1, called presenilin #2, accounts for approximately 25 percent of patients with early-onset Alzheimer's disease.

Chromosome #12 The mutated gene found on this chromosome is believed responsible for 15 percent of late-onset Alzheimer's.

Chromosome #14 The mutated gene on this chromosome, called presenilin #1, accounts for approximately 70 percent of early-onset Alzheimer's.

Chromosome #19 Carries the apolipoprotein E4 gene allele (APOE 4). It also carries apolipoprotein C1, which is also considered a risk factor for Alzheimer's disease The genetic mutation for Down's syndrome is also found here.

Chromosome #21 Known as the Amyloid Precursor Protein (APP) gene, this mutated gene is responsible for approximately 5 percent of familial Alzheimer's disease of the early-onset type.

Chromosomes Thread-like, pared molecules in cell nuclei to which genes are attached. A single chromosome can carry many thousands of genes.

Coenzyme Q10 A molecule found in small amounts in every cell of the body. it enhances the electron transport system (energy transfer) and protects the mitochondria against damage by free radicals.

Creutzfeldt-Jakob Disease A chronic low-grade viral infection, also known as mad cow disease, that attacks the brain and is eventually fatal. Its symptoms are similar to Alzheimer's.

Delusion Mental disorder leading to false and unshakable beliefs.

Dementia A condition marked by memory loss plus a minimum of one other cognitive impairment.

Dementia Pugilistica A dementia common to boxers due to repeated head trauma and, not infrequently, unconsciousness. This dementia can double the incidence of Alzheimer's, and possession of the APOE 4 gene markedly increases incidence tenfold.

DHEA Known as the "mother hormone," it is produced by the adrenal gland and is the precursor of steroids, estrogen, progesterone, and testosterone. Most recent research indicates that it is protective against prostate cancer, but its full impact on Alzheimer's requires more study.

DNA DNA (deoxyribonucleic acid) is a long chainlike structure that is the major component of chromosomes and genes. It is the physical substance of inheritance and is responsible for genetic copying.

Down's Syndrome A genetically-linked hereditary disorder. The abnormal genes for both Alzheimer's and Down's syndrome are found on the same chromosome, #19.

Electromagnetism A strong electrical current with magnetic properties. Evidence is now surfacing indicating that it is a potential cause of Alzheimer's disease.

Electron Transport The flow of energy produced by the mitochondria of every cell in the body. Dysfunctions are responsible for slow nerve degeneration, cellular death, and the progression of Alzheimer's.

Encephalopathy Swelling of the brain caused by many different entities such as trauma and viral or bacterial infection.

Estrogen A female hormone that provides a 55 percent reduction in risk of developing Alzheimer's disease, as well as several other beneficial effects.

Excitotoxin An occurrence in the glutamine neurotransmitting system whereby brain cells become toxic and "excited" which can lead to nerve damage and death.

Fingerprint Patterns They provide markers that can predict the development of Alzheimer's years prior to clinically apparent symptoms of the disease.

Free Radicals Highly reactive molecules that contain an extra electron. They attach themselves to normal body cells such as blood vessels or brain cells and cause damage.

Frontotemporal Dementia Pathology located in the temples and front part of the brain. It causes a dementia nearly identical to Alzheimer's but can be differentiated by MRI scanning. It is clinically differentiated by the loss of inhibitions.

Genes The basic units of heredity, they are comprised of DNA and located on chromosomes.

Ginkgo Biloba An herb that increases circulation to the brain and improves mental performance. It is a free radical scavenger and potent antioxidant.

Ginseng An herb that acts as a mental tonic, increases circulation to the brain, and enhances attention and alertness. It is an immune booster, antioxidant, and free radical scavenger that can improve well-being and sexual drive.

Glutamine An amino acid utilized in a neurotransmitting system.

Gotu Kola An herb that increases circulation to the brain, improves alertness and mental acuity, helps insomnia, and in China is reputed to function as a longevity agent.

Hallucinations A sensory disturbance involving vision and hearing causing an individual to hear or see things that do not exist.

Helicobacter Pylori A bacterium found in the stomach and believed to be responsible for 95 percent of all gastric ulcers. The common housefly is believed to be the host that spreads the bacteria.

Herbal Naturally occurring plant substances such as flowers, bark or roots that are used to treat most known diseases and illnesses.

Herpes Simplex A virus that causes skin or mouth lesions known as fever blisters. It can attack the brain and cause meningitis. If the individual carries the APOE 4 allele, the risk and incidence of developing Alzheimer's disease increases considerably.

Hippocampus A segment of the brain involved with learning and memory and the area most involved with Alzheimer's.

Histamine H$_1$ A substance produced in excess by individuals with allergy and asthma that is responsible for the symptoms.

Histamine H$_2$ A particular type of histamine involved with the production of stomach acid that has no relationship to allergy. It is responsible for chronic inflammation in the brain that, in turn, leads to Alzheimer's. Its activity can be blocked using medicines that are antagonistic to it.

HLA 24 Gene Those who carry this gene develop Alzheimer's two to four years earlier than those who do not.

Hypoglycemia Low blood sugar. It results in nearly double the incidence of Alzheimer's.

Genetics Pertaining to gene-linked inheritance.

Interleukin-6 A chemical that is found in the brain and seen in response to inflammation. Can also be produced due to prolonged physical stress.

Magnetic Resonance Imaging (MRI) Three-dimensional views that avoid X rays and use magnetism. MRI is ninety-five percent accurate in diagnosing Alzheimer's.

Melatonin An amino acid that functions as a hormone, antioxidant, neurotransmitter, free radical scavenger, immune booster, and beta-amyloid blocker. It can help sundowner's syndrome by regulating circadian rhythms.

Meningitis Infection of the brain caused by the herpes simplex virus (meningitis) that will greatly increase the chance of developing Alzheimer's in an individual carrying APOE 4.

Mercury Dental fillings and mercury are implicated as a cause of Alzheimer's. Autopsy studies, however, fail to show a significant increase of brain mercury in Alzheimer's compared to controls.

Microglia A particular type of brain cell that activates to kill off infection but can be maligned and tricked into attacking normal nerve cells and causing damage.

Mini-Stroke Syndrome Multiple small strokes that can eventually lead to dementia.

Muscarinic Receptor A type of cholinergic nerve receptor found in the synapse.

Mutation When an embryonic cell divides and continually doubles in growth, an error may occur in the production of its identical copy, known as a mutation, that then replicates to future generations. A gene can mutate at any age.

Nerve Growth Factor A hormone that promotes the growth of nerve cells in the brain and elsewhere in the body. Experimentally, it has been shown to stimulate the regrowth of new cells in the hippocampal segment of the brains of mice, even after the loss of one-third of their synapses, and to restore functions to normal.

Neurofibrillary Tangles Twisted, damaged, and dead nerve cells secondary to toxic protein plaques and nerve excitotoxicity. Often referred to as "ghosts" and "tombstones."

Neurotransmitter A combination of brain chemicals (amino acids) that transmit nerve impulses across synapses. There are over fifty different neurotransmitters in the brain.

Nicotine A cholinergic stimulator that improves learning and cognition when acting upon the hippocampal brain segment. Receptors to it are found at the synapse.

Nicotinic Receptors Found on nerve cell synapses. They exhibit specific reactions.

Olfactory Lobe A segment of the brain involved with the sensation of smell.

Oxidative Stress A pathological metabolic reaction that causes plaque deposition, neurotoxicity, and diminished energy transfer, all of which can result in neurofibrillary tangles and brain death.

Paranoid Neurotic or psychotic false ideations that people are plotting against them, talking about them, or are intent on doing harm to them.

Pathological Abnormal.

Peptides Molecules that are combinations of amino acids.

PET Scan Positron emission tomography. It is unique for measuring blood flow and glucose utilization, and metabolism of the brain. With three-dimensional views, it is reported as 99 percent accurate in diagnosing Alzheimer's.

Plaquing Clumping of toxic protein between nerve fibers in the brain, leading to cell damage and death.

Presenilin A mutated gene responsible for early onset of disease. Two of these genes have been identified.

Protein Molecules comprised of amino acids. The type in the brain known as amyloid protein can become toxic and form plaques, which in turn adversely affect the neurons and cause cell damage and death. The toxic protein in the plaques is known as beta-amyloid.

SADAS Neuropsychological test known as the Standard Alzheimer's Disease Assessment Scale. It is a battery of several individual tests covering wide areas of ability and is an accurate diagnostic tool.

Schizophrenia A psychosis, or mental illness, often presenting with depression. Symptoms in severe cases can mimic Alzheimer's dementia.

SPECT Scan Single Photon Emission Computed Tomography. It is a three-dimensional model with a 95 percent sensitivity in diagnosing Alzheimer's.

Sundowner's Syndrome A term coined to describe the roaming and wandering of Alzheimer's patients after the sun goes down. It is attributed, in part, to a deficiency of melatonin.

Synapse Connection or junction between two nerve cells. A minuscule space between these nerve endings measuring one billionth of an inch. It contains a neurotransmitter enabling nerve impulses to travel.

Synaptotagmin A protein present in the brain and the cerebrospinal fluid. There is a marked reduction of this protein in the cerebrospinal fluid associated with early onset of Alzheimer's disease.

Synergistic When two entities complement and potentiate one another with a resultant increase in strength or effect.

Tau A protein found in the cerebrospinal fluid. It is present early in the Alzheimer's process in increased amounts.

Thiamine (vitamin B$_1$) A vitamin essential for chemical reactions in the brain. A deficiency in thiamine is found in Alzheimer's dementia, as revealed by autopsy.

3-D MRI Scanner Magnetic resonance imaging via three-dimensional scanning using magnetism instead of X rays. Is 95 percent accurate in diagnosing and in following Alzheimer's by measuring hippocampal atrophy and changes in the temporal lobes.

TIA Transient Cerebral Ischemic Attack. It is a minor brain stroke with either no discernible symptoms or minimal, transitory symptoms. Repeated episodes can lead to brain damage and dementia resembling Alzheimer's.

Tranquilizers A class of drugs designed to reduce anxiety and other nervous disorders.

Tyrosine An amino acid essential for the production of several neurotransmitters including epinephrine (adrenaline). Autopsy reveals deficiencies of tyrosine in Alzheimer's.

Ulnar Loops Fingerprint patterns pointing away from the thumb that act as an early marker to predict Alzheimer's.

Zinc Several recent scientific studies strongly implicate zinc as a potential cause of Alzheimer's.

References

ABRAHAM, A. S. ET AL. 1980. "The Effect of Chromium on Established Atherosclerotic Plaques in Rabbits." *American Journal of Clinical Nutrition* 33(11) (November): 2294–98.

AISEN, P. S. 1996. "Inflammation and Alzheimer's Disease." *Molecular Neuropathology* 28(1) (May–August): 83–88.

AISEN, P. S. ET AL. 1996. "A Pilot Study in Prednisone in Alzheimer's Disease." *Dementia* 7(4) (July–August): 201–6.

AIZAWA, Y. ET AL. 1997. "Amino-terminus Truncated Apolipoprotein E Is the Major Species in Amyloid Deposits in Alzheimer's Disease-Affected Brains: A Possible Role for Apolipoprotein E in Alzheimer's Disease." *Brain Research* 768 (1–2) (September): 208–214.

ANAND, R. ET AL. "Experimental Drug (EXELON™: ENA713)." *Sandoz Pharmeceutical* Online. Internet. Available: http://www.brain net.org/Alz_drugs.htm.

ARMSTRONG, R. A., S. J. WINSPER, AND J. A. BLAIR. 1995. "Hypothesis: Is Alzheimer's Disease a Metal-Induced Immune Disorder?" *Neurodegeneration* 4(1) (March): 107–11.

ARSLAND, D., AND K. LAAKE. 1996. "Should Alzheimer's Disease Be Treated with Tacrine? Review of the Literature." *Tidsskrift For Den Norska Laegeforening* 116(23) (September): 2791–94.

BAGCHI D., M. BAGCHI, AND S. J. STOHS. 1997. "Comparative in Vitro Oxygen Radical Scavenging Ability of Zinc Methionine and Selected Zinc Salts, and Antioxidants." *General Pharmacology* 28(1) (January): 85–91.

BALL, M. J., J. A. KAYE, AND I. STEINER. 1997. "Neocortical Temporal Lobe Sclerosis Masquerading as Alzheimer Dementia: Does Herpes Virus Encephalopathy Protect against Alzheimer's Disease?" *Clinical Neuropathology* 16(1) (January–February): 1–12.

BALLARD, C. ET AL. 1996. "The Prevalence, Associations, and Symptoms of Depression Amongst Dementia Sufferers." *Journal of Affective Disorders* 36(3–4) (22 January): 135–44.

BARCIKOWSKA, M. ET AL. 1995. "Creutzfeldt-Jakob Disease with Alzheimer-type A Beta-reactive Amyloid Plaques." *Histopathology* 26(5) (May): 445–50.

BARNERM, E. L, AND S. L. GRAY. 1998. "Donepezil Use in Alzheimer Disease." *Annals of Pharmacotherapeutics* 32(1) (January): 70–77.

BAUER, J., AND M. HULL. 1995. "Pathogenic Factors of Alzheimer's Disease." *Zeitschrift Fur Gerontologie Und Geriatrie* 28(3) (May–June): 155.

BEAL, M. F. 1996. "Mitochondria, Free Radicals, and Neurodegeneration." *Current Opinion in Neurobiology* 6(5) (October): 661–66.

BEARD, C. M. 1996. "Cause of Death in Alzheimer's Disease." *Annals of Epidemiology* 6(3): 195–200.

BEHL, C. ET AL. 1992. "Vitamin E Protects Nerve Cells from Amyloid Beta Protein Toxicity." *Biochemical Biophysical Research Communications* 186(20) (31 July): 944–50.

BERGMAN, H. ET AL. 1997. "HM-PAO (CERETEC) SPECT Brain Scanning in the Diagnosis of Alzheimer's Disease." *Journal of the American Geriatric Society* 45(1) (January): 15–20.

BIERER, L. M. ET AL. 1995. "Neurochemical Correlates of Dementia Severity in Alzheimer's Disease: Relative Importance of the Cholinergic Deficits." *Journal of Neurochemistry* 64(2) (February): 749–60.

BJERTNESS, E. ET AL. 1996. "Content of Brain Aluminum Is Not Elevated in Alzheimer's Disease." *Alzheimer's Disease and Associated Disorders* 10(3) (fall): 171–74.

BLACKER, D. ET AL. 1997. "APOE 4 and Age at Onset of Alzheimer's Disease: The NIMH Genetics Initiative." *Neurology* 48(1) (January): 139–47.

BLASS, JOHN P. 1996. "Alzheimer's Disease: Melting Pot or Mosaic?" *Alzheimer's Disease Review* 1: 17–20. Online. Available http://www.coa.ukyedu/ADReview/Blass.htm.

BLAYLOCK, R. L. 1996. "Energy-Producing Enzymes and Alzheimer's." *Healthy and Natural Journal* 3(2).

BODICK, N. C. ET AL. 1997. "Effects of Xanomeline, a Selective Muscarinic Receptor Agonist, on Cognitive Function and Behavioral Symptoms in Alzheimer's Disease." *Archives of Neurobiology* 54(4) (April): 465–73.

BORNE, R. F. 1994. "Serotonin: The Neurotransmitter for the '90s." *Drug Topics* (10 October): 108.

BOWEN, J. ET AL. 1997. "Progression to Dementia in Patients with Isolated Memory Loss." *Lancet* 349 (9054) (15 March): 763–65.

BOWLER J. V. ET AL. 1997. "Comparative Evolution of Alzheimer's Disease, Vascular Dementia, and Mixed Dementia." *Archives of Neurology*, Vol. 54: 697–703.

BRAVERMAN, E. R. ET AL. 1997a. "Glutamic Acid." *The Healing Nutrients Within*. Los Angeles: Keats Publishing, Inc.: 239–61.

———. 1997b. "Carnitine." *The Healing Nutrients Within*. Los Angeles, Keats Publishing, Inc.: 366–79.

BREITNER, J. C. ET AL. 1995. "Delayed Onset of Alzheimer's Disease with Non-steroidal Anti-inflammatory and Histamine H_2 Blocking Drugs." *Neurobiology of Aging* 16(4) (July–August): 523–30.

———. 1996. "The Role of Anti-inflammatory Drugs in the Prevention and Treatment of Alzheimer's Disease." *Annual Review of Medicine* 47: 401–11.

BURDETTE, J. H. ET AL. 1996. "Alzheimer's Disease: Improved Visual Interpretation of PET Images by Using Three-dimensional Stereotaxic Surface Projections." *Radiology* 198(3) (March): 837–43.

CAMPION, D. ET AL. 1996. "A Novel Presenilin 1 Mutation Resulting in Familiar Alzheimer's Disease with an Onset Age of 29 Years." *Neuroreport* 7(10) (8 July): 1582–84.

CARNEIRO, R. C., AND R. J. REITER. 1998. "Melatonin Protects Against Lipid Peroxidation Induced by Delta-Aminolevulinic Acid in Rat Cerebellum, Cortex and Hippocampus." *Neuroscience* 82(1) (January): 293–99.

"Cerebrospinal Fluid: A New Biochemical Marker for Synaptic Pathology in Alzheimer's Disease?" *Molecular Chemical Neuropathology* 27(2) (February 1996): 195–210.

CHAKRAVORTY, S. G., AND U. HALBREICH. 1997. "The Influence of Estrogen on Monoamine Oxidase Activity." *Psychopharmacology Bulletin* 33(2): 229–33.

CHAMPION, E. W., ED. 1996. "Editorial: When a Mind Dies." *New England Journal of Medicine* Vol. 334: 791–92.

CHAN, T. Y., AND P. L. TANG. 1995. "Effect of Melatonin on the Maintenance of Cholesterol Homeostasis in the Rat." *Endocrine Research* 21(3) (August): 681–96.

CHANDRA, R. K. 1984. "Excessive Intake of Zinc Impairs Immune Responses." *Journal of the American Medical Association* 252.11 (21 September): 1443–46.

CHEN, L. D. ET AL. 1995. "Melatonin's Inhibitory Effect on Growth of ME-180 Human Cervical Cancer Cells Is Related to Intracellular Glutathione Concentrations." *Cancer Letters* 91(2) (8 May): 153–59.

COLE, M. G., AND J. F. PRCHAL. 1984. "Low Serum Vitamin B_{12} in Alzheimer-type Dementia." *Age Ageing* 13(2) (March): 101–05.

CORRIGAN, F. M. 1991. "Tin and Fatty Acids in Dementia." *Prostaglandins Leukotrienes and Essential Fatty Acids* 43(4) (August): 229–38.

CORRIGAN, F. M. ET AL. 1998. "Abnormal Content of n-6 and n-3 Long-chain Unsaturated Fatty Acids in the Hippocampal Cortex from Alzheimer's Disease Patients." *International Journal of Biochemistry and Cellular Biology* 30(2) (February): 197–207.

———. 1991. "Essential Fatty Acids in Alzheimer's Disease." *Annals of the New York Academy of Science* 640: 250–52.

CRAFT, S., AND J. NEWCOMER. 1996. "Memory Improvement Following Induced Hyperinsulinemia in Alzheimer's Disease." *Neurobiological Aging* 17(1) (January–February): 123–30.

CRAFT, S. ET AL. 1998. "Cerebrospinal Fluid and Plasma Insulin Levels in Alzheimer's Disease." *Neurology* 50(1) (January): 164–68.

CRAWFORD, J. G. 1996. "Alzheimer's Disease Risk Factors as Related to Cerebral Blood Flow." *Medical Hypothesis* 46(4) (April): 367–77.

CROOK, T. ET AL. 1992. "Effects of Phosphatidylserine in Alzheimer's Disease." *Psychopharmacology Bulletin* 28: 61–66.

CRUTS, M., L. HENDRICKS, AND C. VAN BROECKHOVEN. 1996. "The Presenilin Genes: A New Gene Family Involved in Alzheimer's Disease Pathology." *Human Molecular Genetics* 5 Spec. No.: 1449–55.

CRUTS, M., AND C. VAN BROECKHOVEN. 1998. "Presenilin Mutations in Alzheimer's Disease." *Human Mutation* 11(3): 183–90.

CUAJUNGCO, M. P., AND G. J. LEES. 1997. "Zinc and Alzheimer's Disease: Is There a Direct Link?" *Brain Research Review* 23(3) (April): 219–36.

DANENBERG, H. D. ET AL. 1995. "Dehydroepiandrosterone Augments M1-muscarinic Receptor-stimulated Amyloid Precursor Protein Secretion in Desensitized PC12M1 Cells." *Annals of the New York Academy of Science* 77(4) (29 December): 300–03.

DANIELS, W. M. ET AL. 1998. "Melatonin Prevents Beta-Amyloid-Induced Lipid Peroxidation." *Journal of Pineal Research* 24(2) (March): 78–82.

DAVIDSSON, P. ET AL. 1996. "Synaptogen, a Synaptic Vesicle Protein, Is Present in Human Cerebrospinal Fluid: A New Biochemical Marker for Synaptic Pathology in Alzheimer's Disease?" *Molecular and Chemical Neuropathology* 27(2) (February): 195–210.

DEADWYLER, S. ET AL. 1996. "Amaplex (CX516) Has Long Term Effects on Neuronal Function." *Experimental: Cortex Pharmaceuticals.*

DEIBEL, M. A., W. D. EHRMANN, AND W. R. MARKESBERY. 1996. "Copper, Iron, and Zinc Imbalances in Severely Degenerated Brain Regions in Alzheimer's Disease: Possible Relation to Oxidative Stress." *Journal of Neurological Science.* 143(1–2) (November): 137–42.

DE LA MONTE, S. M. ET AL. 1996. "Profiles of Neuronal Thread Protein Expression in Alzheimer's Disease." *Journal of Neuropathology and Experimental Neurology* 55(10) (October): 1038–50.

DE LA TORRE, AND J. V. HACHINSKI. 1996. "Cerebrovascular Pathology in Alzheimer's Disease." *New York Academy of Science Conference* (12–15 November).

DICKSON, D.W. 1998. "Pick's Disease: A Modern Approach." *Brain Pathology* 8(29) (April): 339–54.

EAGGER, S. A. AND R. J. HARVEY. 1995. "Clinical Heterogeneity: Responders to Cholinergic Therapy." *Alzheimer's Disease Associated Disorders* 9(2): 37–42.

EDLAND, S. D. ET AL. 1997. "Increases Risks If Dementia in Mothers of Alzheimer's Disease Cases: Evidence for Maternal Inheritance." *Neurology* 47(1) (July): 245–46.

EDWARDS, R. ET AL. 1998. "Omega-3 Polyunsaturated Fatty Acid Levels in the Diet and in Red Blood Cell Membranes of Depressed Patients." *Journal of Affective Disorders* 48(2–3) (March): 149–55.

ESLER, W. P. ET AL. 1996. "Zinc-Induced Aggregation of Human and Rat Beta-Amyloid Peptides in Vitro." *Journal of Neurochemistry* 66(20) (February): 723–32.

FARRER, L. A. ET AL. 1995. "Rates of Progression of Alzheimer's Disease Is Associated with Genetic Risk." *Archives of Neurology* 52(9) (September): 918–23.

FEKKES, D. ET AL. 1998. "Abnormal Amino Acid Metabolism in Patients with Early Stage Alzheimer's Dementia." *Journal of Neural Transmission* 105(2–3): 287–294.

FITZSIMON, J. S. ET AL. 1997. "Response of the Pupil to Tropicamide Is Not a Reliable Test for Alzheimer's Disease." *Archives of Neurology* 54 (February): 155–59.

FORBES, W. F., AND D. R. MCLACHLAN. 1996. "Further Thoughts on the Aluminum-Alzheimer's Link." *Journal of Epidemiology and Community Health* 50(4) (August): 401–03.

FOX, N. C. ET AL. 1996. "Presymptomatic Hippocampal Atrophy in Alzheimer's Disease. A Longitudinal MRI Study." *Brain* 116 (Part VI) (December): 2001–07.

FRAPE, D. L., AND A. M. JONES. 1995. "Chronic and Postprandial Responses of Plasma Insulin, Glucose and Lipids in Volunteers Given

Dietary Fiber Supplements." *British Journal of Nutrition* 73.5 (May): 733–51.

FROLICH, L., AND P. RIEDERER. 1995. "Free Radical Mechanisms in Dementia of Alzheimer's Type for Antioxidative Treatment." *Arzmeimittelforschung* 45(3A) (March): 443–46.

FUJII, M. ET AL. 1994. "Disorganized Eye Movements and Visuospatial Dysfunctions in an Early Stage of the Patients with Alzheimer's Disease." *Seishin Shinkeigaku Zasshi* 96(5): 357–74.

FULTON, B., AND P. BENFIELD. 1996. "Galanthamine." *Drugs and Aging* 9(1) (July): 60–67.

FUNG, Y. K. ET AL. 1997. "Brain Mercury in Neurodegenerative Disorders." *Journal of Toxicology and Clinical Toxicology* 35(1): 49–54.

GARCIA, J. J. ET AL. 1998. "Melatonin Enhances Tamoxifen's Ability to Prevent the Reduction in Microsomal Membrane Fluidity Induced by Lipid Peroxidation." *Journal of Membrane Biology* 162(1) (1 March): 59–65.

GIRI, S. ET AL. 1998. "Oral Estrogen Improves Serum Lipids, Homocysteine and Fibrinolysis in Elderly Men." *Atherosclerosis* 137(2) (April): 359–66.

GLASKY, A. J. ET AL. 1994. "Effect of AIT-082, a Purine Analog, on Working Memory in Normal and Aged Mice." *Pharmacology Biochemistry and Behavior* 47: 325–29.

GOLD, M., L. A. LIGHTFOOT, AND T. HNATH-CHISOLM. 1996. "Hearing Loss in a Memory Disorders Clinic: A Specially Vulnerable Population." *Archives of Neurology* 53(9) (September): 922–28.

GOLD, M. ET AL. 1995. "Plasma and Red Blood Cell Thiamine Deficiency in Patients with Dementia of the Alzheimer's Type." *Archives of Neurology* 52: 1080–86.

GORDON, G. B. ET AL. 1988. "Reduction of Atherosclerosis by Administration of Dehydroepiandrosterone. A Study in the Hypercholesterolemic New Zealand White Rabbit with Aortic Intimal Injury." *Journal of Clinical Investigations* 82(2) (August): 712–20.

GRANT, W. B. 1997. "Dietary Links to Alzheimer's Disease." *Alzheimer's Disease Review* 2: 42–55.

GRASBY, D. C. 1997. "Pathological Hallmarks of Alzheimer's Disease." Department of Pathology, Clinical School, University of Tasmania, Hobart, Tasmania 7000, Australia. Online. Available: http://werple.mira.net.au/~dhs/paper1.html.

GRAY, C. W., AND A. J. PATEL. 1995. "Neurodegeneration Mediated by Gluta-mate and Beta-amyloid Peptide: A Comparison and Possible Interaction." *Brain Research* 691(1–2) (11 September): 169–79.

GUERRERO, J. M. ET AL. 1997. "Melatonin Prevents Increases in Neural Nitric Oxide and Cyclic GMP Production After Transient Brain Ischemia and Reperfusion in the Mongolian Gerbil (Meriones Unguiculatus)." *Journal of Pineal Research* 23(1) (August): 24–31.

GUO, Q. ET AL. 1997. "Alzheimer's Presenilin Mutation Sensitizes Neural Cells to Apoptosis Induced by Trophic Factor Withdrawal and Amyloid Beta-peptide: Involvement of Calcium and Oxyradicals." *Journal of Neuroscience* 17(11) (1 June): 4212–22.

HALBREICH, U. ET AL. 1995. "Estrogen Augments Serotonergic Activity in Postmenopausal Women." *Biological Psychiatry* 37(7)(1 April): 434–41.

HAMPSON, R. E. ET AL. 1998. "Facilitative Effects of the Ampakine CX516 on Short-Term Memory in Rats: Correlations with Hippocampal Neuronal Activity." *Journal of Neuroscience* 18(7) (1 April): 2748–63.

HENDERSON, V. W., L. WATT, AND J. G. BUCKWALTER. 1996. "Cognitive Skills Associated with Estrogen Replacement in Women with Alzheimer's Disease." *Psychoneuroendocrinology* 21(4) (May): 421–30.

HENDLER, SHELDON S. ET AL. 1990. *The Doctors' Vitamin and Mineral Encyclopedia*. New York, NY: Fireside, Simon & Schuster.

HEROUX, M. ET AL. 1996. "Alterations of Thiamin Phosphorylation and of Thiamin-Dependent Enzymes in Alzheimer's Disease." *Metabolic Brain Disorders* 11.1 (March): 8198.

HIGAKI, J., G. M. MURPHY, AND B. CORDELL. 1997. "Inhibition of Beta-Amyloid Formation by Haloperidol: A Possible Mechanism for Reduced Frequency of Alzheimer's Disease Pathology in Schizophrenia." *Journal of Neurochemistry* 68 (1) (January): 333–36.

HILL, E. G., S. B. JOHNSON, AND R. T. HOLMAN. 1979. "Intensification of Essential Fatty Acid Deficiency in the Rat by Dietary Trans Fatty Acids." *Journal of Nutrition* 109(10) (October): 1759–65.

HILLER, R. ET AL. 1995. "Serum Zinc and Serum Lipid Profiles in 778 Adults." *Annals of Epidemiology* 6 (November): 490–96.

HIRASHIMA, N. ET AL. 1996. "Calcium Responses in Human Fibroblasts: A Diagnostic Molecular Profile for Alzheimer's Disease." *Neurobiology of Aging* 17(4) (July–August): 549–55.

HOBBS, CHRISTOPHER. 1996. *The Ginsengs: A User's Guide*. Santa Cruz, CA: Botanica Press.

HOOPER, P. L. ET AL. 1980. "Zinc Lowers High-Density Lipoprotein-Cholesterol Levels." *Journal of the American Medical Association* 244(17) (October): 1960–61.

HORN, R. ET AL. 1996. "Atrophy of the Hippocampus in Patients with Alzheimer's Disease and Other Diseases with Memory Impairment." *Dementia* 7(4) (July–August): 182–86.

HULL, M. ET AL. 1996a. "Interleukin-6-Associated Inflammatory Processes in Alzheimer's Disease: New Therapeutic Options." *Neurobiology of Aging* 17(5) (September–October): 795–800.

———. 1996b. "The Participation of Interleukin-6, a Stress-inducible Cytokine in the Pathogenesis of Alzheimer's Disease." *Behavioral Brain Research* 78(1) (June): 37–41.

ISHII, K. ET AL. 1996. "The Clinical Utility of Visual Evaluation of Scintigraphic Perfusion Patterns for Alzheimer's Disease." *Clinical Nuclear Medicine* 21(2) (February): 106–10.

ITAGAKI, T. ET AL. 1996. "Glucose Metabolism and Alzheimer's Disease." *Nippon Ronen Igakkai Zasshi* 33(8) (August): 569–72.

ITZHAKI, R. F. ET AL. 1997. "Herpes Simplex Virus Type 1 in Brain and Risk of Alzheimer's Disease." *Lancet* 349(9047) (January): 241–314.

JENDROSKA, K. ET AL. 1995. "Ischemic Stress Induces Deposition of Amyloid Beta Immunoreactivity in Human Brain." *Acta Neuropathologica* 90(58): 461–6.

JOOSTEN, E. ET AL. 1997. "Is Metabolic Evidence for Vitamin B_{12} and Folate Deficiency More Frequent in Elderly Patients with

Alzheimer's Disease?" *Journal of Gerontology and Biological Science* 52(2) (March): M76–79.

JORDAN, B. D. ET AL. 1997. "Apolipoprotein E Epsilon 4 Associated with Chronic Traumatic Brain Injury in Boxing." *Journal of the American Medical Association* 278(2) (2 July): 136–40.

JOST, B. C., AND G. T. GROSSBERG. 1996. "The Evolution of Symptoms in Alzheimer's Disease. A Natural History Study." *Journal of the American Geriatric Society* 44(9) (September): 1078–81.

KALARIA, R. N. 1996. "Cellular Aspects of the Inflammatory Response in Alzheimer's Disease." *Neurodegeneration* 4(5) (December): 487–503.

KAWAS, C. ET AL. 1997. "More Proof That Estrogen Replacement May Be Effective Against Alzheimer's." *Neurology* (June): 1517–21.

KEIMOWITZ, R. M. 1997. "Dementia Improvement with Cytotoxic Chemotherapy. A Case of Alzheimer's Disease and Multiple Myeloma." *Archives of Neurology* 54(4) (April): 485–88.

KEISSLING, L., AND R. MURPHY. 1997. "Toxic Protein Discovery May Lead to New Understanding of Alzheimer's." *Meeting of the American Chemical Society* (14 April).

KENNARD, M. L. ET AL. 1996. "Serum Levels of the Iron Binding Protein Are Elevated in Alzheimer's Disease." *Nature Medicine* 2(11) (2 November): 1230–35.

KHOO, S. K., AND P. CHICK. 1992. "Sex Steroid Hormones and Breast Cancer: Is There a Link with Oral Contraceptives and Hormone Replacement Therapy?" *Medical Journal of Australia* 156(2) (20 January):124–32.

KITAGAKI, H. ET AL. 1997. "Alteration of White Matter MR Signal Intensity in Frontotemporal Dementia." *American Journal of Neuroradiology* 18(2) (February): 367–78.

KLIVENYI, P., AND L. VESCEI. 1997. "Neurodegeneration: Aging and Dementia. Etiopathogenic Role of Electron Transport Disorders." *Orvosi Hetilap* 138(6) (9 February): 331–35.

KUKULL, W. A. ET AL. 1995. "Solvent Exposure as a Risk Factor for

Alzheimer's Disease: A Case-control Study." *American Journal of Epidemiology* 141(11) (1 June): 790–1059.

KURZ A., R. MARQUARD, AND D. MOSCH. 1995. "Tacrine: Progress in Treatment of Alzheimer's Disease." *Zeitschrift Fur Gerentologie und Geriatrie* 28(3) (May): 163–68.

LAUTENSCHLAGER, N. T. ET AL. 1996. "Risk of Dementia Among Relatives of Alzheimer's Disease Patients in the Mirage Study: What Is in Store for the Oldest Old?" *Neurology* 46(3) (March): 641–50.

LAWRENCE, A. D., AND B. J. SAHAKIAN. 1995. "Alzheimer's Disease, Attention, and the Cholinergic System." *Alzheimer's Disease and Associated Disorders* 9 Suppl. 2: 43–49.

LENDON, C. L., F. ASHALL, AND A. M. GOATE. 1997. "Exploring the Etiology of Alzheimer's Disease Using Molecular Genetics." *Journal of the American Medical Association* 227(10) (March): 825–31.

LEVY, M. L. ET AL. 1996. "Alzheimer's Disease and Frontotemporal Dementias. Behavioral Distinctions." *Archives of Neurology* 53(7) (July): 687–90.

———. 1997. "Alzheimer's Disease and Frontotemporal Dementia." *Archives of Neurology* 54. (April): 350.

LIN, W. R., D. SHANG, AND R. F. ITZHAKI. 1996. "Neurotropic Viruses and Alzheimer's Disease. Interaction of Herpes Simplex Type 1 Virus and Apolipoprotein E in the Etiology of the Disease." *Molecular Chemical Neuropathology* 1(3) (May–August): 135–41.

LOCKE, P. A. ET AL. 1995. "Apolipoprotein E4 Allele and Alzheimer's Disease: Examination of Allelic Association and Effect on Age at Onset in Both Early and Late-onset Cases." *Genetic Epidemiology* 12(1): 83–92.

LOPEZ, O. L. ET AL. 1995. "Computed Tomography—But Not Magnetic Resonance Imaging—Identified Periventricular White-matter Lesions Predict Symptomatic Cerebrovascular Disease in Probable Alzheimer's Disease." *Archives of Neurology* 52(7) (July): 659–64.

LYKETSOS, C. G. ET AL. 1996. "Guidelines to the Use of Tacrine in Alzheimer's Disease: Clinical Application and Effectiveness." *Journal of Neuropsychiatry and Clinical Neuroscience* 8(1) (Winter): 67–73.

MAHIEUX, F. ET AL. 1995. "Isoform 4 of Apolipoprotein E and Alzheimer Disease. Specificity and Clinical Study." *Revue Neurologique* 151(4) (April): 231.9.

MAO, X., AND S. W. BARGER. 1998. "Neuroprotection by Dehydro-epiandosterone-sulfate: Role of an NfkappaB-like Factor." *Neuroreport* 9(4) (9 March): 759–63.

MASTERS, C. ET AL. 1997. "Alzheimer's Disease Research." Online. Available: http://www.mhri.edu.au/adr. 26 June.

MASTROGIACOMA, F. ET AL. 1996. "Brain Thiamine, Its Esters, and Its Metabolizing Enzymes in Alzheimer's Disease." *Annals of Neurology* 39(5) (May): 585–591.

MAURIZI, C. P. 1995. "The Mystery of Alzheimer's Disease and Its Prevention by Melatonin." *Med. Hypotheses* 45(4) (October): 339–40.

MAYEUX, R. ET AL. 1998. "Utility of the Apolipoprotein E Genotype in the Diagnosis of Alzheimer's Disease." *The New England Journal of Medicine* 338(8) (19 February): 506–11.

McCADDON, A. ET AL. 1998. "Total Serum Homocysteine in Senile Dementia of Alzheimer Type." *International Journal of Geriatric Psychiatry* 13(4) (April): 235–39.

McGEER, P. L., AND E. G. McGEER. 1996. "Anti-inflammatory Drugs in the Fight Against Alzheimer's Disease." *Annals of the New York Academy of Science* 777 (17 January): 213–20.

———. 1995. "The Inflammatory Response System of the Brain: Implications for Therapy of Alzheimer's and Other Neurodegenerative Diseases." *Brain Research Reviews* 21(2) (September): 195–218.

MECKS, J. 1997. "U.S. Faces Healthcare Crisis." Online. Available: http://www.alz.org/assoc/media/natrl.htm.

MENDEZ, M. F. ET AL. 1996. "Frontotemporal Dementia Versus Alzheimer's Dementia: Differential, Cognitive Features." *Neurology* 47(5) (November): 1189–94.

MENTIS, M. J. ET AL. 1996. "Visual Cortical Dysfunction in Alzheimer's Disease with a Graded 'Stress Test' During PET." *American Journal of Psychiatry* 153(1): 32–40.

MIDDLEMISS, P. J. ET AL. 1995. "AIT-082, a Unique Purine Derivative, Enhances Nerve Growth Factor Mediated Neurite Outgrowth from PC 12 Cells." *Neuroscience Letters* 199: 1–4.

MILLER, T. P. ET AL. 1998. "Cognitive and Non-Cognitive Symptoms in Dementia Patients: Relationship to Cortisol and Dehydroepiandrosterone." *International Psychogeriatrics* 10(1) (March): 85–96.

MIMORI, Y., H. KATSUOKA, AND S. NAKAMURA. 1996. "Thiamine Therapy in Alzheimer's Disease." *Metabolic Brain Disease* 11(1) (March): 89–94.

MING-XIN, T. ET AL. 1998. "The APOE 4 Allele and the Risk of Alzheimer's Disease Among African-Americans, Whites and Hispanics." *Journal of the American Medical Association* 279 (11 March): 751–55.

MOLSA, P. K., R. J. MARTTILA, AND U. K. RINNE. 1995. "Long-Term Survival and Predictors of Mortality in Alzheimer's Disease and Multi-infarct Dementia." *Acta Neurologica Scandanaviea* 91(3) (March): 159–64.

MORDENTE, A. ET AL. 1998. "Antioxidant Properties of 2, 3-dimethoxy-5-methyl-6-(10-hydroxydecyl)-1, 4-benzoquinone (Idebenone)." *Chemical Research in Toxicology* 11(1) (January): 54–63.

MORGAN, C. D., S. NORDIN, AND C. MURPHY. 1995. "Odor Identification as an Early Marker for Alzheimer's Disease: Impact of Lexical Functioning and Detection Sensitivity." *Journal of Clinical Experiments in Neuropsychology* 17(5) (October): 793–803.

MORI, E. ET AL. 1997. "Premorbid Brain Size as a Determinant of Reserve Capacity Against Intellectual Decline in Alzheimer's Disease." *American Journal of Psychiatry* 154(1) (January): 18–24.

MORTIMER, J. A. 1995. "Continuum Hypothesis of Alzheimer's Disease and Normal Aging: The Role of Brain Reserve." *Alzheimer's Research* 1(2) (August): 67–70.

MOWREY, DANIEL B. 1986. *The Scientific Validation of Herbal Medicine.* New Canaan, CT: Keats Publishing, Inc.

MYERS, D. H. ET AL. 1996. "Apolipoprotein E Epsilon 4 Association with Dementia in a Population-based Study: The Framingham Study." *Neurology* 46(3) (March): 673–77.

NICOLL, J. A., G. W. ROBERTS, AND D. I. GRAHAM. 1996. "Amyloid Beta Protein, APOE Genotype and Head Injury." *Annals of the New York Academy of Science* 7779 (17 January): 271–75.

NIELSEN, F. H. ET AL. 1994. "Biochemical and Physiologic Consequences of Boron Deprivation in Humans." *Environmental Health Perspectives* 102 Suppl. 7 (November): 59–63.

NORMAN, J. ET AL. 1995. "Apolipoprotein E Genotype and Its Effect on Duration and Severity of Early and Late Onset Alzheimer's Disease." *British Journal of Psychiatry* 167(4) (October): 533–36.

OBENBERGER, J., AND J. ROTH. 1995. "Selegiline in the Treatment of Alzheimer's Disease." *Neurologicka* 134(12) (June): 388–90.

OKEN, R. J. 1995. "Antihistamines, A Possible Risk Factor for Alzheimer's." *Medical Hypothesis* 44(1) (January): 47–48.

ORGOGOZO, J. M. ET AL. 1997. "Wine Consumption and Dementia in the Elderly: A Prospective Community Study in the Bordeaux Area." *Revue Neurologique* (Paris) 153(3) (April): 185–92.

PAGANINI-HILL, A. AND V. W. HENDERSON. 1996. "Replacement Therapy and Risk of Alzheimer's Disease." *Archives International Medicine* (28 October) 156(19): 2213–17

PARKER, W. D., AND R. E. DAVIS. 1997. "Large Subset of Alzheimer's Cases May Be Maternally Inherited." *Proceedings of the National Academy of Sciences.* (29 April).

PAYAMI, H. ET AL. 1996. "Gender Difference in Apolipoprotein E-associated Risk for Familial Alzheimer's Disease: A Possible Clue to the Higher Incidence of Alzheimer's Disease in Women." *American Journal of Human Genetics* 58(4) (April): 803–11.

PEDERSEN, W. A. ET AL. 1996. "Amyloid Beta-protein Reduces Acetylcholine Synthesis in a Cell Line Derived from Cholinergic Neurons of the Basal Forebrain." *Proceedings of the National Academy of Sciences* 93–15 (23 July): 8068–71.

PERICAK-VANCE, M. A. ET AL. 1997. "Complete Genomic Screen in Late-Onset Familial Alzheimer's Disease." *Journal of the American Medical Association* 278 (15 October): 1237–41.

PHILLIPS, H. ET AL. 1997. "NGF May Provide a Key to Reversing the Effects of Alzheimer's." *Doctors Guide to Medical and Other News* (2 October).

PLOTNICK, G. D. ET AL. 1997. "Effect of Antioxidant Vitamins on the Transient Impairment of Endothelial-Dependent Brachial Artery Vasoconstriction Following a Single High Fat Meal." *Journal of the American Medical Association* 278 (11 December): 1635–1716.

PODUSLO, S. E. ET AL. 1995. "A Closely Linked Gene to Lipoprotein E. May Serve as an Additional Risk Factor for Alzheimer's." *Neuroscience Letters* 201(1) (December): 81–83.

RASMUSSEN, D. X. ET AL. 1995. "Head Injury as a Risk Factor in Alzheimer's Disease." *Brain Injury* 9(3) (April): 213–19.

REIMAN, R. ET AL. 1996. "Preclinical Evidence of Alzheimer's Disease in Persons Homozygous for the (Epsilon) 4 Allele for Apolipoprotein E." *New England Journal of Medicine* 334(12) (21 March): 752–58.

REITER, R. J. 1995a. "Oxygen Radical Detoxification Processes During Aging: The Functional Importance of Melatonin." *Aging* 7(5) (October): 340–51.

————. 1995b. "The Pineal Gland and Melatonin in Relation to Aging: A Summary of the Theories and of the Data." *Experimental Gerontology* 30(3–4) (May–August): 199–212.

REITER, R. J., R. C. CARNEIRO, AND C. S. OH. (1997) "Melatonin in Relation to Cellular Antioxidative Defense Mechanisms." *Hormone and Metabolic Research* 29(8) (August): 363–72.

RICH, J. B. ET AL. 1995. "Nonsteroidal Anti-inflammatory Drugs in Alzheimer's Disease." *Neurology* 45(1) (January): 51.5.

RIEKKINEN, P., JR. ET AL. 1995. "Hippocampal Atrophy, Acute THA

Treatment and Memory in Alzheimer's Disease." *Neuroreport* 6(9) (19 June): 1297–3000.

RIEMENSCHNEIDER, M. ET AL. 1997. "Diagnosis of Alzheimer's Disease with Cerebrospinal Fluid Tau Protein and Aspartate Aminotransferase." *The Lancet* 350(9080) (13 September).

RIPA, S., AND R. RIPA. 1994a. "Zinc and Atherosclerosis." *Minerva Medica* 85(12) (December): 647–54.

———. 1994b. "Zinc and Arterial Pressure." *Minerva Medica* 85(9) (September): 455–59.

———. 1995. "Zinc and Immune Function." *Minerva Medica* 86(7–8) (July–August): 315–18.

ROGERS, J. 1995. "Inflammation as a Pathogenic Mechanism in Alzheimer's Disease." *Arzeneimittelfirschung* 45.3A (March): 439–42.

ROGERS, S. L. ET AL. 1998. "Donepezil Improves Cognition and Global Function in Alzheimer's Disease: A 15-week, Double-Blind, Placebo-controlled Study. Donepezil Study Group." *Archives of Internal Medicine* 158(9) (11 May): 1021–31.

ROGERS, S. L., AND L. T. FRIEDHOFF. 1996. "The Efficacy and Safety of Donepezil in Patients with Alzheimer's Disease: Results of a U.S. Multicenter, Randomized, Double-Blind, Placebo-controlled Trial." *Dementia* 7(6) (November–December): 293–303.

ROSENBERG, R. N. ET AL. 1996. "Genetic Factors for the Development of Alzheimer's Disease in the Cherokee Indian." *Archives of Neurology* 53(10) (October): 997–1000.

ROSES, A. D. 1996a. "Apolipoprotein E Alleles as Risk Factors in Alzheimer's Disease." *Annual Review of Medicine* 47: 387–400.

———. 1996b. "Apolipoprotein E and Alzheimer's Disease. A Rapidly Expanding Field with Medical and Epidemiological Consequences." *Annals of the New York Academy of Science* 802 (December): 50–57.

———. 1997. "Genetic Testing for Alzheimer's." *Archives of Neurology* 54 (October): 1226–29.

ROSLER, N. ET AL. 1996. "Dementias—Diagnosis, Differential Diagnosis, and Therapy." *Fortschritte Der Medizen* 114(28) (10 October): 351–56.

SANDBRINK, R. ET AL. 1996a. "Genes Contributing to Alzheimer's Disease." *Molecular Psychiatry* 1(1) (March): 27–40.

———. 1996b. "USF Develops New Cell Transplant Technology." *Biotechnology* 14(3): 1692–95.

SANO, S. M. ET AL. 1970. "A Controlled Trial of Selegiline, Alpha-tocopherol, or Both as Treatment for Alzheimer's. The Alzheimer's Disease Cooperative Study." *New England Journal of Medicine* 336(17) (24 April): 1216–22.

SASTRE, J. ET AL. 1998. "A Ginkgo Biloba Extract (EGb 761) Prevents Mitochondrial Aging by Protecting Against Oxidative Stress." *Free Radical Biology and Medicine* 24(2) (15 January): 298–304.

SCHELLENBERG, G. D. 1995. "Genetic Dissection of Alzheimer Disease, A Heterogeneous Disorder." *Proceedings of the National Academy of Science* 92(19) (12 September): 8552–59.

SCHENK, D. ET AL. 1997. "The PDAPP Transgenic Mouse as an Animal Model for A-beta-induced Amyloidosis and Neuropathology." *Alzheimer's Disease Review* 2: 20–27.

SCHOTT, K. ET AL. 1996. "Antibody Reactivity in Serum of Patients with Alzheimer's Disease and Other Age-related Dementias." *Psychiatry Research* 59(3) (31 January): 251–54.

SCOTT, W. K. ET AL. 1997. "Apolipoprotein E Epsilon 2 Does Not Increase Risk of Early-onset Sporadic Alzheimer's Disease." *Annals of Neurology* 42(3) (September): 376–78.

SIU, A. W., R. J. REITER, AND C. H. TO. 1998. "The Efficacy of Vitamin E and Melatonin as Antioxidants Against Lipid Peroxidation in Rat Retinal Homogenates." *Journal of Pineal Research* 24(4) (May): 239–44.

SMALL, G. ET AL. 1997. "Alzheimer's Disease Onset Time Linked to HLA-2A." *Neurology* 49: 512–17.

SMITH, M. A., AND G. PERRY. 1995. "Free Radical Damage, Iron, and Alzheimer's Disease." *Journal of Neurological Science* 134 Suppl (December): 92–94.

SMITH, M. A., L. SAYRE, AND G. PERRY. 1996. "Is Alzheimer's a Disease of Oxidative Stress?" *Alzheimer's Disease Review* 1: 63–67.

SNOWDON, D. A. 1996. "Linguistic Ability in Early Life and Cognitive Function and Alzheimer's in Late Life: Findings from the Nun Study." *Journal of the American Medical Association* 275(7) (21 February): 528–32.

SOBEL, E., ET AL. 1995. "Occupations with Exposure to Electromagnetic Fields: A Possible Risk Factor for Alzheimer's Disease." *American Journal of Epidemiology* 142(5) (September): 515–24.

———. 1996. "Elevated Risk of Alzheimer's Disease Among Workers with Likely Electromagnetic Field Exposure." *Neurology* 47 (6) (December): 1477–81.

SOLOMON, A. R. ET AL. 1996. "Nicotine Inhibits Amyloid Formation by the Beta-peptide." *Biochemistry* 35(42) (October): 13568–78.

SOLOMON, P. R. ET AL. 1998. "Recognition of Alzheimer's Disease: The 7-Minute Screen." *Family Medicine* 30(4) (April): 265–77.

STANDISH, M. I. ET AL. 1996. "Improved Reliability of the Standardized Alzheimer's Disease Assessment Scale (SADAD) Compared with the Alzheimer'sDisease Assessment Scale (ADAS)." *Journal American Geriatric Society* 44(6) (June): 712–16.

STERN, Y., ET AL. 1997. "Predicting Time to Nursing Home Care and Death in individuals with Alzheimer's Disease." *Journal of the American Medical Association* 227(10) (March): 806–12.

STEWART, W. F. ET AL. 1997. "Risk of Alzheimer's Disease and Duration of NSAID." *Neurology* 48(3) (March): 626–32.

STUSS, D. T. ET AL. 1966. "Do Long Tests Yield a More Accurate Diagnosis of Dementia Than Short Tests?" *Archives of Neurology* 53 (October): 1033–39.

SUGAYA, E. ET AL. 1997. "Nervous Diseases and Kampo (Japanese herbal) Medicine: A New Paradigm of Therapy Against Intractable Nervous Diseases." *Brain Development* 19(2) (March): 93–103.

SVENSSON A. L., AND A. NORDBERG. 1998. "Tacrine and Donepezil Attenuate the Neurotoxic Effect of A-beta (25–35) in Rat PC 12 Cells." *Neuroreport* 9(7) (11 May): 1519–22.

TAGLIALATELA G., ET AL. 1996. "Spatial Memory and NGF Levels in Aged Rats: Natural Variability and Effects of Acetyl-L-Carnitine Treatment." *Experimental Gerontology* 31(5) (September): 577–87.

TANABE, J. L. ET AL. 1997. "Tissue Segmentation of the Brain in Alzheimer's Disease." *American Journal of Neurology* 18(1) (January): 115–23.

TANG, M. X. ET AL. 1996. "Effect of Age, Ethnicity, and Head Injury on the Association Between APOE Genotypes and Alzheimer's Disease." *Annals of the New York Academy of Sciences* 802 (December): 6–15.

TEUNISSE, S. ET AL. 1996. "Dementia and Subnormal Levels of Vitamin B_{12}: Effects of Replacement Therapy on Dementia." *Journal of Neurology* 243(7) (July): 522–29.

THOME, J. ET AL. 1997. "Oxidative Stress Associated Parameters in Serum of Patients with Alzheimer's Disease." *Life Science* 60(1): 13.9.

TIERNEY, M. C., ET AL. 1996. "Prediction of Probable Alzheimer's Disease in Memory-impaired Patients: A Prospective Longitudinal Study." *Neurology* 46(3) (March): 661–65.

TOGHI, H. ET AL. 1994. "Concentrations of Alpha-tocopherol and Its Quinone Derivative in Cerebrospinal Fluid from Patients with Vascular Dementia of the Binswanger Type and Alzheimer Type Dementia." *Neuroscience Letters* 174(1) (6 June): 73–76.

TOLBERT, S. R., AND M. A. FULLER. 1996. "Selegiline in the Treatment of Behavioral and Cognitive Symptoms of Alzheimer's Disease." *Annals of Pharmacotherapy* 30(10) (October): 1122–29.

TROJANOWSKI, J. 1997. "New Plaque Protein Identified in Brains of People with Alzheimer's." *American Journal of Pathology* 151: 69–80.

VAN DUIJN, C. M. ET AL. 1995. "The Apolipoprotein E Epsilon 2 Allele Is Associated with an Increased Risk of Early-onset Alzheimer's Disease and a Reduced Survival." *Annals of Neurology* 37(5) (May): 605.10.

VAN GOOL, W. A. 1995. "Diagnosing Alzheimer's Disease in Elderly, Mildly Demented Patients: The Impact of Routine Single Photon Emission Computed Tomography." *Journal of Neurology* 242(6) (June): 401–05.

WAKABAYASHI, S. 1992. "The Effects of Indigestible Dextrin on Sugar Tolerance: I. Studies on Digestion-Absorption and Sugar Tolerance." *Nippon Naibunpi Gakkai Zasshi* 68(6) (20 June): 623–35.

WALKER, JOHN, AND Z. KMIETOWICZ, EDS. 1997. "Nobel Prize Winners Unravel Aging Process." *British Medical Journal* 7115 (315) (25 October).

WATSON, R. R. ET AL. 1996. "Dehydroepiandrosterone and Diseases of Aging." *Drugs and Aging* 9(4) (October): 274–91.

WEINROB, H. 1985. "Fingerprint Patterns in Alzheimer's Disease." *Archives of Neurology* 42: 50–54.

WHITEHOUSE, P. J., AND R. N. KALARIA. 1995. "Nicotinic Receptors and Neurodegenerative Dementing Diseases: Basic Research and Clinical Implications." *Alzheimer's Disease Association Disorders* 9(2): 3–5.

WILSON, A. L. ET AL. 1995. "Nicotinic Patches in Alzheimer's Disease: Pilot Study on Learning, Memory, and Safety." *Pharmacology, Biochemistry, and Behavior* 51 (2–3) (June–July): 509–14.

XANTHAKOS, S. ET AL. 1996. "Magnetic Resonance Imaging of Alzheimer's Disease." *Progress for Neuropsychopharmacology and Biological Psychiatry* 20(4) (May): 597–626.

XU, S. AND F. GASKIN. 1997. "Increased Incidence of Anti-Beta Antibodies Secreted by Epstein-Barr Virus Transformed B Cell Lines from Patients with Alzheimer's Disease." *Mechanisms of Aging Development* 94 (1–3) (March): 213–22.

YAN, S. D. ET AL. 1996. "RAGE and Amyloid-beta Peptide Neurotoxicity in Alzheimer's Disease." *Nature* 328.6593 (August): 685–91.

YANASE, T. 1996. "Serum Dehydroepiandrosterone (DHEA) and DHEA-sulfate (DHEA-S) in Alzheimer's Disease and in Cerebrovascular Dementia." *Endocrinology* 43(1) (February): 119–23.

YOSHIDA, H., AND F. YOSHIMASU. 1996. "Alzheimer's Disease and Trace Elements." *Nippon Rinso* 54(1) (January): 111–16.

ZAMAN, Z. ET AL. 1992. "Plasma Concentrations of Vitamins A and E and Carotinoids in Alzheimer's Disease." *Age and Aging* 21(20) (March): 91–94.

ZUBENKO, G. S. ET AL. 1996. "Premorbid History of Major Depression and the Depressive Syndrome of Alzheimer's Disease." *American Journal of Geriatric Psychiatry* Vol. 4: 85–90.

Index